Cured to Death

Cured to Death

The Effects of Prescription Drugs

Arabella Melville and Colin Johnson

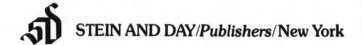 STEIN AND DAY/*Publishers*/New York

First published in the United States of America in 1983
Copyright © 1982 by Arabella Melville and Colin Johnson
All rights reserved
Printed in the United States of America

STEIN AND DAY / *Publishers*
Scarborough House
Briarcliff Manor, N.Y. 10510

Library of Congress Cataloging in Publication Data

Melville, Arabella, 1948-
    Cured to death.

    Bibliography: p.
    Includes index.
    1. Drugs—Side effects.   2. Drugs—Toxicology.
3. Iatrogenic diseases.   4. Medicine—Philosophy.
I. Johnson, Colin, 1939-   II. Title.
[DNLM: 1. Drugs and narcotic control.   2. Drug
industry.   3. Drug therapy—Adverse effects.   4. Drug
therapy—Utilization.   WB 330 M531c]
RM302.5.M44   1983   615.5'8   82-42523
ISBN 0-8128-2889-5

Contents

Acknowledgements

We cannot acknowledge all the people who have given generously of their time and resources to contribute parts of the jigsaw puzzle from which this book grew.

However, we are particularly indebted to the following: Roy Mapes, Professor of Sociology, University College of Swansea, for guidance over wide areas and invaluable practical help; John McKinlay, Professor of Sociology, Boston University; Jean Trainor and members of the Eraldin Action Group, Birmingham; Bryn Williams and Merthyr Tydfil Community Health Council; Sid Wolfe, Ben Gordon, and the Public Citizen Health Research Group, Washington, DC; Arthur Levin and the Centre for Medical Consumers, New York City; Richard Crout and members of the FDA staff, especially Judy Jones; Jo Hodgson for support and help with typing. For painstaking editorial work on the final typescript, we thank Rivers Scott.

Lastly, we cannot quantify the contribution made by Peter Grose throughout the many stages of this book's metamorphosis, from early discussion of the idea to publication.

A Note on Terminology

The terminology of the medical industry is a tangle of fine distinctions, rough definitions and implied meanings. The medical profession adds to popular confusion by using a language which excludes patients from discussion or understanding. In addition, there are international variations within the terminological morass.

Throughout this book, we have whenever possible used the most commonly accepted terms to convey the meaning simply. Where this has not been possible, or where the term in question has many meanings, we hope that clarity will emerge from the context. This note is intended as a foundation for readers who are unfamiliar with the subject

1 DRUGS

Any substance which alters the state of body or mind is, in the widest sense, a *drug*.

It can be a single entity, that is, a simple *chemical substance*, or a *biological product*. A medicine may contain a combination of various drug ingredients.

The majority of available drugs are *synthetic*, that is, they are either a manufactured copy of a naturally occurring substance, or, more usually, an artificially created substance that would not normally occur in nature.

Where we use the term drug it refers to a substance normally only available on a *prescription* issued by a qualified person, such as a doctor or dentist, who is a *licensed medical practitioner*.

Prescription drugs are also called *ethical drugs*, or *ethical pharmaceuticals*.

Other medicinal drugs are classified as *non-prescription, proprietary* or *over-the-counter* (OTC) drugs. Although these drugs may be prescribed, they can be sold directly to the public and are advertised in the same way as any other consumer product.

2 DRUG NAMES

The naming of drugs is a complex subject. Each drug will have at least three sorts of name. These are: the chemical name, the generic name and the brand name.

The *chemical name* is a description of the molecular structure of the drug, and only of interest to chemists. The *generic name* is an agreed shortened form of the chemical name, which gives some clue to the type of chemicals involved. The *brand*, or *trade*, *name* is the name the drug manufacturer uses for the product.

Whereas the generic name for the substance will usually be the same all over the world, the same substance may have a different brand name in every country, or even more than one brand name if more than one company produces it.

For example: The hydrochloride of 7-chloro-4-dimethylamino-1,4,4a,5, 5a,6,11,12a-octahydro-3,6,10,12,12a-pentahydroxy-6-methyl-1,11-dioxo-2-napthacene carboxamide is the *chemical* name referring to chlortetracycline hydrochloride, the *generic name* of the drug which has Aureomycin as the *brand name* registered by American Cyanamid.

In this book we use both generic and brand names. Brand names are given with capital initial letters, thus: Penbritin; and generic in lower case, thus: ampicillin.

3 DRUG EFFECTS

Those effects which may be considered *beneficial* or *therapeutic* include the relief of pain, the modification of a body process, the altered perception of a stimulus, the elimination of unwanted or harmful organisms, the replacement of vital process intermediaries, or any combination of these.

Side effects of drugs are any effects other than the intended therapeutic effects which occur at normal therapeutic doses. They are not necessarily dangerous or unpleasant.

Adverse drug reactions (ADRs) are the noxious, unintended and usually unpredictable effects of drugs. They can vary in seriousness through mild skin rashes to permanent body damage or death.

4 DRUG MANUFACTURERS

The commercial companies who make and sell prescription drugs refer to themselves as *pharmaceutical manufacturers*, or *producers of ethical pharmaceuticals*, and collectively as the *pharmaceutical industry*, or the *ethical pharmaceutical industry*.

Drug manufacturers are frequently large *multinational corporations*, with subsidiaries in many parts of the world.

5 MISCELLANEOUS TERMS

Any pharmaceutical product is classed as *ethical* if it is advertised only to members of the medical profession.

When a drug manufacturer develops a new drug it may be protected by a *patent*. This is an internationally recognised *legal monopoly* granted by governments for a number of years. A company with a patented drug may *license* other companies to manufacture and sell the drug, in return for the payment of *royalties*.

Part One

A Bitter Pill

"The requirements of health can be stated simply. Those who are fortunate enough to be born free of significant congenital disease or disability will remain well if three basic needs are met. They must be adequately fed; they must be protected from a wide range of hazards in the environment; and they must not depart radically from the pattern of personal behaviour under which man evolved — for example by smoking, over-eating, or sedentary living."

Thomas McKeown, The Role of Medicine

Chapter One

Consider the Possibility

This book makes a definite statement. It is this: Western medicine has made a fundamental error in allowing itself to become reliant on the universal use of drug therapy.

It is an error both of philosophy and of tactics. Our examination of the effects of prescription drugs on patients, doctors and the institutions of health care has led us inevitably to this conclusion. Our statement runs counter to accepted wisdom, contradicts many popularly held beliefs and is contrary to the ideology and motivation of some of the largest and most powerful industrial interests in the world. We are convinced that the evidence is irrefutable and cannot be interpreted in any other way. We ask you to consider the possibility that drugs, rather than helping or curing, are actually doing harm.

It is true that through vaccination, some infectious diseases can be eradicated; that drugs provide effective therapy for previously fatal conditions; and that analgesia and anaesthesia make life more bearable. The problem is one of perspective. Drugs have become the predominant force in health care, to the detriment of other approaches.

The spectacular beginning of the modern drug age may blind us to the fact that *all* drugs, whatever their virtues, are inherently dangerous.[1] The nature of the substances that the pharmaceutical industry produces is such that, inevitably, unforeseen disasters will happen. Thalidomide and practolol have been recent examples. With the exception of the personal suffering, the most important effect of these tragedies has been that the essential nature, attitudes and priorities of the pharmaceutical manufacturers were revealed to a wide critical audience.[2] This insight forced those governments which had not previously done so to accept the need for some degree of control over the activities of drug manufacturers, and to monitor the uses to which their products were put.

Nevertheless, potential for further disaster remains. It arises from the nature of the organisations which assess, manufacture and promote drugs, from the way they are prescribed and from our attitudes to medicine.

Before delving into the details of these complexities, we must lift the layer of public relations imagery that has been carefully drawn over drugs and their use in our society.

It is easy to forget that the pharmaceutical industry, with its endless multiplicity of products and world-wide multi-billion-dollar turnover, is a phenomenon of the last forty years. Most of the discoveries that have made the world significantly safer pre-date it, and drugs which made the most important contributions to human well-being were available before the industry developed. The British Pharmacopoea of 1932 contained just 36 synthetic drugs, including aspirin, phenacetin and barbitone, all of which had been developed in Germany before 1900.[3] In the United States an examination of the two hundred most frequently dispensed drugs in the late 1960s showed that only five had been introduced during the nineteenth century, five between 1900 and 1929 and nine in the 1930s.[4]

Drugs are manufactured by commercial organisations for the same reasons as any other product: to make a profit. The primary reason for the existence of any incorporated business is to benefit its shareholders. Drug companies make money by selling drugs.

Different countries have different rules and regulations concerning the way drugs are sold to doctors and pharmacists and attempt to control an industry known for selling as hard and fast as possible. Each part of every potential market is subjected to some of the most intensive sales promotion the world has known. From invention to market, a new drug can cost a company a decade's work and tens of millions of dollars. At that price you cannot afford to admit to many mistakes.

Nevertheless mistakes do happen, even after the lesson of thalidomide, and most governments now accept that drug manufacturers cannot be given complete freedom to sell whatever drugs they choose. Most parts of the world now have some form of regulatory agency to control drug marketing and to assess the risks of drug use among their populations. These regulatory bodies range from the American Food and Drugs Administration (FDA), which is fairly effective, through the bureaucratic deference of the British Committee on Safety of Medicines (CSM), to those which are simply window dressing.

People rely on doctors, both to protect them from exposure to drug hazards and to prescribe appropriate medicine. In the opinion of one influential English physician, 'Prescribing works in a sufficient number of cases to encourage both doctor and recipient to think they must be on the right track. . . It is so mechanistic a half-trained sheepdog could do it and you would hardly notice the difference in most cases.'[5]

It is generally accepted that the vast majority of primary care consultations, perhaps as many as 90 per cent, are not about treatable medical problems. Yet in the UK, more than three quarters of all consultations end with a prescription for drugs, and in some countries the proportion approaches 100 per cent. Doctors everywhere have developed habits of unnecessary, inappropriate or frankly dangerous prescribing. In much of the third world even the inadequate protection provided by the nominal supervision of the physician may be lacking, for potent medicines intended for specialised use and available elsewhere on prescription only, are sold like sweets or candy over the counter to anyone.

If drug therapy is being so misused, why are its dangers not well known? Perhaps because we assume drugs do good, and we fail to question our beliefs. Drug monitoring is not considered important. There are also serious practical problems; drugs are consumed in such enormous quantities that monitoring their real effects is a gigantic task. If a particular drug becomes suspect, word of serious adverse effects is expected to filter through the medical journals to warn doctors to take more care. The regulatory agencies set up to provide protection lack teeth. Even governments have found that they must tread carefully when confronting the pharmaceutical industry, as the West German government found when it withdrew marketing permission for ICI's clofibrate in the late 1970s. The company promptly threatened legal action against the government and in a short time the drug was available again for use in West Germany.[6] This was despite the evidence of a comprehensive clinical trial which showed that the drug caused more harm than good.[7]

People who run drug companies are 'not bishops, they are businessmen',[8] to quote one of their English spokesmen. And they act accordingly with considerable success; their businesses worldwide are at the top of profit, growth and award tables. Consequently they are popular with shareholders and governments alike. This popularity causes problems when the same governments wish to exert their role as guardians of public interest by controlling them.

Under a veneer of cooperation and goodwill, the drug industry is constantly fighting to extend its spheres of influence. The penetration of the fabric of government, the medical profession, academic and research institutions and the mass media is extensive.[9] In most industrial countries, though they try to maintain a low profile, the drug manufacturers are among the most powerful political and economic pressure groups.[10]

The thrusting spirit at the core of the pharmaceutical industry has encouraged it to extend its operations from the manufacture and marketing of cures, into the forward marketing areas, where it is actively discovering conditions that can be promoted as illnesses. Doctors are routinely advised on the necessary treatment for such conditions as 'restless legs'. However unlikely the ill, the industry will be able to provide the appropriate pill.

Despite their power and riches, drug companies are the rawest nerve of the medical care industry. All would protest vehemently that their endeavours are vital, and indisputably contribute to the general well-being. But is this true? Is the almost unrestricted dominance of drug therapy in medicine acceptable?

Any examination of the state of sickness, health and death among the population in the developed countries raises fundamental doubts that cannot be explained in terms of isolated tragic episodes. Belief in the curative power of drugs has shifted emphasis and diverted resources away from the positive promotion of health. Despite the enormous growth of the drug bill, clear benefit cannot be demonstrated. The money spent has no effect on the broad determinants of health in a community, and frequently other cost-effective treatments are restricted for lack of money. Under the aegis of universal chemotherapy, medicine is no longer practised: it is administered.

In a world context the most effective general health measure would be the provision of adequate clean water. The sale of a range of esoteric drugs not only masks real problems; it squanders the resources needed for basic provisions.

As a result of the way prescription drugs are used, iatrogenic disease – literally 'doctor-caused' disease, but now most commonly disease caused by drugs – is an enormous and growing medical problem. When it appears, the usual answer is to prescribe the unfortunate victim yet another drug, with its own hazards, for the new symptoms. Even under the specialised care of hospitals, perhaps as many as 28 per cent of patients suffer adverse reactions to their medication.[11]

Drug-induced disease leads to many deaths. In both the United States[12] and Britain it has been calculated that more people are killed each year by prescribed drugs than by accidents on the roads. The figures for the maimed and injured may be proportionately higher. There is no reason to believe that this level of casualties does not occur in every country where pharmaceutical products are widely used.

Drug-induced deaths occur predominantly among the older or more feeble members of the population, and because of this the cause of death will be obscured. But with the growth in the use of drugs for more and more everyday conditions, iatrogenic disease is emerging as a clear entity. As society increases its dependence on drugs, iatrogenic disease becomes the consequence we have to live and die with.

The most common public debate about drugs concerns their price.

From our perspective, this has the air of a sponsored irrelevance. If a drug were able to cure a disease and save lives it might be priceless, but whether a certain type of tablet is very cheap or incredibly expensive is not the point that should be under discussion. Of paramount importance is the effect of that drug when used over a long period on massive numbers of people. Drugs which cause even small amounts of iatrogenesis can rapidly incur cost penalties. The subsequent treatment and care of the victims of drugs that may have cost pennies can rapidly run into tens or hundreds of thousands of pounds. In 1970 Dr Donald Brodie, of the National Center for Health Services Research and Development, stated that the annual cost of adverse reactions in the United States was in excess of $1 billion.[13] And no price can ever be put on the human misery and despair involved.

The traditional role of the physician has been dramatically distorted by the ready availability of potent drugs, and the power-base of his position has moved from the social and healing arts to his control over the prescription pad. It is understandable that doctors should seek easy answers. Theirs is an impossible task. But reliance on drugs has not provided any real answers, let alone easy ones. It has merely created another impossible situation for the doctor. Every year brings a new crop of drugs which he is taught about by the self-interested drug companies. If he is to prescribe with any appropriate degree of care he must keep up to date. With perhaps 25,000 drugs in various forms, simply knowing what is available may be impossible. When you add to this the rate at which information is produced, it can be seen that the attempt is hopeless. The British Monthly Index of Medical Specialities (MIMS) in November 1980 noted 80 deleted products; 43 additional forms of existing drugs; 41 deleted forms; 47 changes in dosage; 26 changes in therapeutic indications; 21 changes in warnings on special precautions; and 69 new products.

The physicians' inability to cope is revealed in the prescriptions they write. In many cases the drugs selected are determined by the doctor's attitudes, not by his patients' conditions or needs.[14] Doctors have an irrational freedom to prescribe that is underwritten by the ancient idea that medicine is an art as well as a science, and art does not require reason. It is expressed in the concept of clinical judgement, which the doctor uses and in which patients have faith. However, doctors are as much victims of prejudice and habit as the rest of us. They too are only human.

The emergence of iatrogenic disease can be too much for the relationship between doctor and patient. The discovery will often produce a reaction of guilt, and the destruction of trust can make sympathetic care impossible. The frustrating and unsatisfactory relationship with doctors has led drug victims to turn to others with similar problems to seek strength and comfort through mutual support. There are growing numbers of such groups organised around a particular condition or concerned with the effects of a particular drug.

Our efforts to maintain health may be based on totally inappropriate assumptions and practices simply because, in the widest context, we lack understanding of the basic natural history of the diseases and ailments which afflict us. The pharmaceutical explosion has not resulted in longer and healthier lives. After thirty years' experience, is the best we can offer the less fortunate nations a means of taking longer to die?

Would it not be the ultimate in tragic irony if our misunderstanding and gross misuse of chemical technology were to conspire against us? Despite the best intentions of the medical industry and the regulatory agencies, it is possible that a drug with potential for massive latent genetic damage, or capable of producing a virulent resistant pathogen, could precipitate the next universal impact of horror on our collective awareness. Such a self-induced plague of white death could make the medieval Black Death pale to insignificance by comparison.

Chapter Two

Seduced by an Idea

There have always been occasions of stress or celebration when it has been thought desirable to alter the perception of reality with drugs. The West traditionally chose alcohol, the East marijuana or opium. Most recently, the social happenings of the late 1960s made an entire generation aware of the possibilities, if not the realities, of illegal drug use. The cross-cultural experimentation with marijuana, opium derivatives and cocaine was extended to great numbers of people, and the widespread use of LSD added to the established repertoire of those seeking escape or modified perception.

Yet whatever one may feel about the use or abuse of illegal substances, they are not the real problem. The picture of the typical drug addict with a dangerous habit must be redrawn, away from long-haired youths or social inadequates and towards ordinary people in the street, who are convinced they are ill and believe they are being cured. Today's drug addict is the person next to you on the bus or in the shop, your colleague at work, your friend. And, increasingly, it is likely to be you who depends on drugs.

How has this alarming situation arisen? It is not something that can be attributed to any group in isolation. Patients, after all, rely almost completely on the medical expertise of doctors. Doctors, over-worked and in the front line of health care, almost invariably respond by prescribing drugs when consulted.[1] They have been led to believe that this is the only way they can cope with the demands made upon them, and they are convinced that it is good for their patients.

Along with the hospital, the doctor is the part of the vast medical care industry of which we are most aware. And behind the doctor, with his superior education, are a variety of institutions, each one contributing its own part of the modern drug jigsaw. These vary from the doctor's professional association, to research facilities, welfare agencies, drug manufacturers and government departments. Each is responsible for providing some part of the medical care facilities that patients wish to call on in time of need.

To each the use of drugs offers an attractive expedient; it enables immediate needs to be satisfied, and offers hope to sufferers from any unwanted condition, while at the same time avoiding the need to question disease causes too deeply. In his day-to-day behaviour the doctor represents the practical effects of a single idea upon all the health care institutions.

This seductive idea, on which modern medical treatment is predominantly based, is that of a German chemist, Paul Ehrlich. In 1906, while working with arsenic compounds in efforts to treat syphilis, he elaborated the concept of a *magic bullet*. In Ehrlich's mind the bullet was a chemical which would kill parasites within the body, and the magic would be the chemical's ability to select the parasite and ignore the host. He said:

> If we picture an organism as infected by a certain species of bacterium, it will obviously be easy to effect a cure if substances have been discovered which have an exclusive affinity for those bacteria and act deleteriously or lethally on these and on these alone, while, at the same time, they possess no affinity whatever for the normal constituents of the body, and cannot therefore have the least harmful, or other, effect on the body. Such substances would then be able to exert their full action exclusively on the parasite harboured within the organism, and would represent, so to speak, *magic bullets* which seek their target of their own accord.[2]

Ehrlich quickly realised the limitations of his original idea. The medical, chemical and pharmaceutical industries did not. Seduced by its powerful simplicity, they have clung to it tenaciously, its attractiveness allowing them to behave as if the necessary prerequisites for its success were indeed established.

In Ehrlich's day the battle against disease was seen as fairly straightforward. There were good guys and bad guys, and it was felt that once appropriate answers were found the bad guys among the organisms would be despatched. Although with the passage of years the picture of illness and disease has become more complex, modern treatments still rely on that earlier, simplistic approach.

Consequently, among modern drugs, some may be considered to have more magic, or be better aimed, than others. Antibiotics are generally highly effective against specific infections, although the body's own defence systems are improved by increased living standards and higher nutritional levels.

But the concept of the carefully aimed bullet can easily degenerate into the casual lobbing of a speculative hand grenade. For example, in the case of atherosclerosis, if the blood vessels are becoming choked with fatty deposits so that blood is impeded in its progress to the hands and feet, what sort of specific 'bullet' would work? One which would strip the fat from the walls of the arteries? At present the type of drug which may be used under these circumstances is one which causes the blood vessels near the surface of the body to dilate. Such an irrelevant and generalised effect is far removed from Ehrlich's original concept.

To understand why the magic bullet is a severely limited idea we must consider in some detail the way drugs work within the body. Drugs are chemical substances which in comparatively small quantities alter the state of the body or mind. All medicines contain drugs, and so incidentally do everyday things like tea, coffee, beer and tobacco. Defining something as a drug does not determine the way in which it is used. Those drugs defined and used as medicines are selected because it is thought that they possess useful properties for treatment of unwanted conditions.

Most drugs act by either stimulating or depressing particular bio-chemical or physiological functions within the body. That is, they change the body's chemistry, usually in complex and subtle ways. Precisely how or why they work are in many cases questions at the frontiers of our knowledge, and complete answers are often far beyond.

For ease of identification and use, drugs are generally divided into 'therapeutic groups' – that is, the substances are grouped according to the particular type of disease they are predominantly used to treat. The number of groups can be as great as the number of diseases or drugs available, but in practice around eighty types are usually identified.

Whilst some of these drugs can be used to combat life-threatening disease, this is rare. In the vast majority of cases they are not essential; sometimes they are totally unnecessary, and frequently they are positively harmful. Yet very few drugs are therapeutically useless. Their value, or lack of it, lies in the way they are used. Later in this book we shall examine the factors which affect the choice of drugs, and which remove most use of medicine from any idea of rational therapy.

Medicines can be swallowed, injected, applied directly to body tissues, inhaled, or inserted as pessaries; but whatever the route into the body, they will not have more than very limited local effects until they enter the blood-stream. The faster a drug reaches the blood-stream, the sooner it is likely to produce its effect. Drugs such as some anaesthetics, which are injected directly into veins, act very quickly, in contrast with drugs which are swallowed and absorbed gradually through the lining of the stomach and intestines.

Drugs circulate with the blood to every part of the body except, in some cases, the brain, which is protected by a special filter known as the blood-brain barrier. When they reach the liver, most drugs are metabolised, or broken down into simpler molecules, and returned to the circulation. Finally, they are eliminated from the body via the kidneys as waste products dissolved in urine.

It is easier to understand drug action if the body is regarded as an electro-chemical machine, operating through a series of chemical reactions which can produce minute electrical charges. The complex chemicals which make up the tissues of the body are constantly interacting with each other, and one function of the blood-stream is to bring fuel for these chemical reactions.

The majority of drugs act by binding to specific sites of body tissues known as receptors. The chemical structure of the drug determines its effect at a particular receptor site. Ehrlich likened this to fitting a special key into a well-designed lock. When a single molecule of the appropriate drug reaches this receptor site it will modify the chemical reaction which takes place there. The few exceptions include drugs such as antacids, which do not generally pass through the walls of the digestive tract but act locally to neutralise stomach acid, and drugs such as germicides which act in a non-specific way to kill living organisms. Some general anaesthetics, too, act in non-specific ways which do not seem to involve combination with specific receptors.[3]

Many drugs are structurally related to naturally occurring molecules and their effects will be similar to those of the natural chemical; but the points of difference can be crucial. They may, for instance, bind to receptor sites for slightly longer than the molecules the sites were designed to fit; and while the drug molecule clings to the receptor, it makes it inaccessible to the natural chemical. Sometimes the drug becomes part of a chemical chain which then stops growing because of the discrepancy. Cytotoxic (anti-cancer) drugs are used in this way to check the multiplication of malignant cells; the drug disrupts the growth of all body tissues, including the tumour.

In the search for new drugs, scientists often look for abnormalities in body chemistry that are associated with illness. For example, it was discovered that depressed people had, on average, lower levels of certain brain chemicals involved in the transmission of nerve impulses than their more cheerful fellows. So drugs were developed which were capable of reducing the rate of breakdown of these transmitter chemicals, thus causing them to accumulate. For the patient, the result is usually an improvement in mood.

Very slight modifications to drug molecules will usually give them markedly different effects. Many natural chemicals are made up of asymmetrical molecules which come in right- and left-handed forms, and it is not unusual for pharmacologists to find that whereas one form produces some dramatic effect, its mirror image will not. LSD is one of the best known of such drugs; only the right-handed, or dextro, form has any effect at all.

Established drugs are often modified in the hope of improving their action. When ICI developed practolol, it was derived from their established drug propranolol. They hoped that slight changes in the structure of propranolol would eliminate its main drawback, a tendency to precipitate bronchospasm in susceptible patients. ICI's scientists were successful; the company was able to claim that practolol was more cardioselective than propranolol. It was only after years of use that the new drug was found to produce adverse effects much more dangerous than bronchospasm, effects which are not shared by propranolol.

The fact that drugs act at specific receptor sites does not mean that Ehrlich's magic bullets have been found. The particular types of natural chemical which are capable of interacting with a given drug are likely to be found in various different types of body tissue and organs. A drug cannot discriminate between different locations of the same receptor, and an action that lacks this sort of specificity is bound to entail dangers.

The predominant effect of a drug is partly dependent on its concentration in the body. Pharmacologists describe the changes in drug effects with increasing doses as dose-response relationships, and they can normally find a series of different dose-response curves for each drug. Occasionally, more than one response can be used in therapy, which is why low doses of a drug may be given for one condition and higher doses for another; for example, the major tranquillizer chlorpromazine (Thorazine, Largactil) may be used in small doses to prevent nausea and vomiting or in high doses to control schizophrenia. More often, the drug effects which predominate at higher doses are unwanted, and the useful therapeutic dose takes account of the level at which these adverse effects occur.

One aim of the extensive testing of new drugs is to find optimum ranges of different therapeutic doses, a problem which is complicated by individual variability in response. One characteristic of a safe drug — as far as any drug can be described as safe – is that the difference between the therapeutic and toxic doses is very large.

On average, a heavier person will need more of a drug to achieve the same effect than will a lighter individual, but the effects of the same dose, whether therapeutic or noxious, also varies independently of body weight. People at extremes of age, both old and young, tend to be more sensitive, and men may differ from women. Illness, eating patterns and any drugs taken concurrently, further complicate the problem. In everyday experience, we know we don't all get predictably drunk on exactly the same quantity of whisky, and medicines can be quite as unpredictable as alcohol.

Metabolism and excretion of drugs prevent their accumulation to dangerous levels in the body during a course of treatment. Anything that interferes with the efficiency of the liver or the kidneys will therefore increase the risk of drug levels building up and of the adverse reactions that occur at high doses. Elderly kidneys are often less efficient than normal at eliminating drugs from the body, and liver damage will tend to reduce the rate of drug metabolism. So a higher concentration of the drug can result from a normal dose given to an old person, causing him to suffer from chronic drug toxicity which may gradually become more severe as treatment continues.

Toxic reactions caused by acute drug overdose are seldom due to exaggeration of the therapeutic effect. In overdose the less preferred and undesirable effects of the drug become dominant, producing damage which may be irreversible.[4] Overdose deaths due to narcotic drugs or barbiturates, for example, are usually the result of depression of the centre of the brain that controls breathing; while paracetamol overdose kills through liver damage.[5]

What about antidotes to drug overdose? Dr Jekyll and Mr Hyde developed the illusion to perfection; in the film you could actually see the antidote working. Although antidotes have a long literary pedigree, they are mainly the products of fantasy. A specific antidote is available in less than two per cent of poisoning cases.

As the authoritive *Prescribers' Journal* puts it: 'Only very rarely is a true pharmacological antagonist, or antidote, available (for overdose cases) and treatment is therefore based on symptomatic and supportive measures.'[6] Damage due to drugs cannot generally be reversed because tissue damage frequently occurs which can only be repaired by the body's own replacement mechanisms over a period of time. This is useless against acute poisoning or overdose.

Nevertheless, the theory of the antidote is so attractive that until very recently it was widely accepted by the medical profession. If, it was argued, a patient had taken an overdose of hypnotics, particularly barbiturate sleeping pills, one could counter the effects by giving the patient stimulant drugs. Two overdoses, as it were, for the price of one. It was only in the early 1960s that a specialised centre in Copenhagen demonstrated that death rates were doubled when stimulant drugs were given in such cases, and provided the medical profession with evidence of the folly of this practice.[7] The administration of drug 'antidotes' is believed to have declined, though not disappeared. It is part of the seductive nature of the treatment that relinquishment of even fatal procedures is painfully difficult for doctors.

Potentiation – where the effects of one drug are exaggerated by the presence of another – is a frequent ally of lethal overdose. As increasing numbers of people rely on poly-drug therapy it is a growing problem, for potentiation is likely when two drugs have a similar effect. It can happen that the combination does not increase the preferred effect of one drug, but boosts a much less desirable side-effect in an unpredictable way.

In the liver, where the majority of the drug will be broken down, one substance may cause a significant decrease in activity, thus allowing dangerous levels of unmetabolised drug to accumulate. The complex problem of how drugs work is immeasurably compounded by the possibilities of interaction, as there are many more variables involved. Serious problems of interaction often cannot be predicted; they are learned by experience.

Antagonism, the opposite of potentiation, is not so serious unless the patient depends on a particular drug to stay alive. Any substance that upsets the enzyme system of the liver can cause antagonism. Tobacco smoke, for instance, speeds up some breakdown processes through 'enzyme induction'. In consequence, the drug is excreted faster, reducing its concentration in the blood-stream, and thus its effect. Simple mechanical interference can also cause antagonism, as when one substance prevents the body from taking up another. For example, milk of magnesia, taken for indigestion, prevents the absorption of the antibiotic tetracycline through the gut.[8]

A substantial proportion of drugs will interact with each other. Usually they act in ways that do not have serious consequences, as when cough mixture and antihistamines are mixed to produce a good, if unexpected, sleeping draught. But other reactions can lead to death, as when anti-coagulants and the anti-rheumatic phenylbutazone are mixed, causing haemorrhage into the body tissues.[9]

Drugs can interact at their sites of action within the body, and if the primary action at that site is not understood, then it is even less likely that any interaction can be predicted or understood.

Obviously the doctor must tread warily through this labyrinth of dangerous complexity when prescribing. The physician William Withering wrote in 1787, when defining the use of foxglove extract, digitalis, in the treatment of heart disorders: 'Poisons in small doses are the best medicines; and useful medicines in too large doses are poisonous.'[10] He might also have added that when poisons are used therapeutically, they should, unless it is absolutely unavoidable, be used one at a time.

Two fundamental questions are raised for patients by the nature of drugs and the way they act. The first is the question of consent to treatment, and the second is that of acceptable risk. Consent is relatively easy to deal with; in practical terms, we have become so used to being given a prescription for drugs whenever we visit the doctor that it no longer arises. If you ask your doctor to treat you for a particular complaint, consent to whatever he decides is implied by your acceptance of the instruction to 'take as directed', whatever the final outcome.

Because of this, the concept of acceptable risk becomes crucial. At the heart of any consideration of risk is the question of the toxic dose and the difference between this and the normal therapeutic dose. For casually used drugs like tranquillizers, the difference should be, and usually is, very large, whereas for drugs given to treat otherwise fatal conditions the difference can obviously be much smaller. For some drugs, Valium for instance, there is no definite lethal dose. With others the lethal dose can be so near the therapeutic that special care must be taken with their use at all times.

With every drug there is a risk, and once we accept the prescribed treatment the risk is unavoidable. Obviously, more risk is acceptable when drugs are used to treat potentially fatal illness. High risk anti-cancer drugs are only used because the alternative, unrestricted growth of the tumour, is dreadful and predictable. Most cytotoxic drugs would be fatal if taken for more than a very short period, often only a matter of weeks, and such risk is clearly only justifiable under extreme circumstances.

Take the case of Judith Carson, a patient with breast cancer. After a mastectomy, her doctors began treatment with the cytotoxic drug uracil mustard. After each course of injections, she was too weak to leave her bed; she was vomiting and aching all over, and oppressed by a sense of deep gloom. At intervals blood samples were taken to check the level of white cells, because uracil mustard causes serious bone-marrow depression. White cells from the bone marrow fight infections, and without them the body's defence systems fail. By accepting the treatment, Judith was risking life-threatening disease, although at the time neither she nor her doctors were aware of any further cancer. They took the risk of treatment with a drug that is both extremely unpleasant to take and very dangerous because the risk posed by the possibility of any tumour cells remaining was considered too serious to ignore.

For both doctors and patients, considered judgements about drug risks require high levels of knowledge of the likely dangers and benefits of treatment. As the available information is continually changing with time and experience, the boundaries of acceptability change for each drug. When it was thought that oral contraceptives were only very rarely associated with thrombosis, stroke and other serious cardiovascular hazards, the risk was generally disregarded. As information accumulated, it became clear that the rise in probability of some sort of cardiovascular disease is enormous, especially for women over thirty-five and those who smoke. For oral contraceptive users the risk of stroke, for example, has been found to be twenty-six times the risk for women of a similar age who do not use the Pill.[11] Publicity about the risks of oral contraception led many women to decide for themselves that the benefits did not justify the risk involved.[12]

Usually, patients are ignorant of the real dangers of the drugs they take. They are content to leave the judgement of risk to the doctor, and many health professionals believe that patients are not capable of judging the hazards involved in the use of medicines. In prescribing, the doctor effectively takes the decision for the patient, and this act precludes consideration of any other form of treatment.

Judgement of risk is largely a matter of perspective. Given the option, most patients are prepared to accept a sliding scale of risk, where the possibility of adverse drug reactions is balanced against the perceived seriousness of the illness. In the majority of his cases the physician is likely to judge risk not in terms of the possibility of cure for the patient, but by whether the drug is a reasonably safe palliative. From their actions it is clear that some drug companies consider an acceptable risk to be anything for which they are not likely to suffer.

Finally, questions of risk must be seen against the general background of drug use in medicine. Patients demand cures for any real or imagined condition, and the reservoir of 'illness' expands to fill the capacity to care for it. Politically, medically and commercially the easiest way to increase the capacity to cope with demand is by the use of more drugs.

Paradoxically, physicians are grossly undereducated in areas associated with drugs, and they are not given the scientific background necessary to evaluate claims made for them. Consequently they rely heavily on the information supplied to them by the drug manufacturers, who are neither unbiased nor objective.[13]

It cannot be stated too often that for a drug to have effect it *must* also have dangers. But, this does not mean that the more dangerous a drug is the more effective it will be.

Any unwanted effects that a drug produces can be classed as adverse reactions. They vary from the unpleasant, typified by the dry mouth produced by most antidepressants, through the tragic like that produced by thalidomide, to the fatal, such as the peculiar form of sclerosing peritonitis caused by practolol.

Three types of adverse reactions are intrinsic properties of drugs. These are side-effects, secondary effects and toxic effects. Every drug can have side-effects at therapeutic doses, although not everyone will be aware of them. They usually occur because the drug action is more general than one would wish: the 'magic bullet' cannot be aimed. The drug is present throughout the body when its effect is only required in a part of it; effects on systems where the drug was not needed are side-effects. If a hay-fever sufferer takes an antihistamine pill it will suppress the action of histamine not only in the nose and sinuses but also in the brain, causing the side-effect of drowsiness. Hay-fever sufferers do not usually need their brain chemistry altered; drowsiness can be a hazard, for instance when driving.

Secondary effects are indirect consequences of drug action. Antibiotics kill bacteria indiscriminately, the good as well as the bad. Bacteria in the gut, respiratory tract and vagina usefully keep down the levels of fungi which otherwise thrive in these warm damp environments. After antibiotic therapy, yeasts (thrush) may proliferate unchecked and cause immense irritation. It can take many months for the natural flora to re-establish itself.[14]

The case of Joan Mills, a sufferer from ulcerative colitis, is a grim example. The treatment for her disease involved long-term steroid drugs (prednisolone). After eight months she developed a dry cough and a fever. She was taken to hospital but died within three days. At the autopsy it was found that she had actually died of tuberculosis. The steroid medication had suppressed the body's immune response which had protected her from recurrence of the tuberculosis from which she had suffered nearly fifty years before. In this case tuberculosis was a secondary effect of the steroid medication.

Toxic effects are due to a direct action of the drug. They usually occur at high dose levels, but they may also happen at normal doses in sensitive individuals. Toxic effects of drugs usually result in tissue damage, such as that to the liver caused by an overdose of paracetamol, or to the auditory nerve by streptomycin, gentamycin and closely related antibiotics. Once initiated, drug damage to the liver or kidneys can obviously produce a spiral of escalating toxic effects.

Most serious adverse drug reactions are well-documented risks of familiar drugs.[15] The commonest symptom is skin rash,[16] which may not in itself seem serious; in most cases, it clears up when the drug responsible is withdrawn. However, drug rashes can warn of greater dangers.

An allergic reaction to a drug often shows initially as a skin rash. Subsequent exposure to the same drug can cause severe illness requiring emergency help. At worst, the result can be death through anaphylactic shock. About twenty people are reported to die from anaphylactic shock caused by penicillin each year in Britain.[17] This is the main drawback of this otherwise remarkably safe and effective drug, and the reason that we are so often asked about allergies when our medical histories are taken.

Anaphylactic shock occurs when a foreign protein is given to a person who has become sensitised to it. Proteins are highly complex molecules which are universally present in living matter. Some drugs are proteins, while others can combine with proteins in the body to form molecular complexes. The body has defence mechanisms which are specifically designed to cope with harmful foreign protein invaders, such as bacteria;

antibodies combine with the invader and they are broken down and ingested by white blood cells.

Unfortunately, the body may not be able to discriminate between noxious bacteria and useful drugs. The relatively enormous quantity of drug circulating throughout the body can precipitate a reaction in every blood vessel at once. This leads to a massive fall in blood pressure, severe asthma, shock and death, unless oxygen and intensive emergency treatment are immediately available.[18] Such tragedies should be, and generally are, avoided by taking heed of previous signs of allergy to that drug.

Until the first signs appear, allergic reactions cannot usually be predicted. They are idiosyncratic reactions to the foreignness of the drug rather than to any specific properties it may possess.

Drug industry spokesmen may try to convey the impression that all adverse drug reactions are idiosyncratic and therefore essentially due to some peculiarity of the victim. However, while it is true that it is usually impossible to predict precisely who will be susceptible, the rate at which such reactions occur may be discovered. For example, it is known[19] that one person in 20,000 who takes the antibiotic chloramphenicol will develop a potentially fatal aplastic anaemia, and many other drugs also have a level of idiosyncratic fatality that is considered acceptable.

For practolol, an outline of the idiosyncratic mechanism that led to the development of the characteristic syndrome of adverse reactions has been pieced together. It appears to have triggered a unique form of immune response, because it was capable of binding to body proteins in such a way that the body reacted to them as foreign. But practolol did not produce anaphylactic shock; its effect was to induce the body to seal off particular sites with scar tissue.[20]

Alan Brown knows he was lucky to survive the effects of practolol. He was put on a maintenance course of the drug after a heart attack. Within a year he developed a body rash, with dry cracking skin on his hands, knees and feet. Tears ran uncontrollably down his face; then they suddenly stopped and his eyes became permanently dry. Severe abdominal pains followed, and his condition rapidly deteriorated. 'My stomach was so bad,' he said, 'that I couldn't keep any food down, I was vomiting within an hour of a meal. I lost three stone. When they operated, I thought I was just going to die, it was that bad.' The surgeons found that Mr Brown had masses of fibrous scar-like tissues strangling his intestines and internal organs. Their diagnosis confirmed that the cause was the unique and dreadful adverse effect of practolol, sclerosing peritonitis.

Adverse reactions of this sort are rare, unpredictable and largely inexplicable. Unfortunately this is true of many serious adverse reactions to drugs.

The body has many interacting functions and systems. Adverse reactions can be caused by the fact that it is impossible to achieve a desired alteration in one body system without producing changes in others. A comparatively straightforward example is the contraceptive pill. By changing sex hormone levels it causes changes in the brain centres which control the natural production of these hormones, and these changes seem to be linked in turn with modifications to the chemical systems which are important in influencing a person's mood. In susceptible women these changes have been implicated in migraine and depression.[21]

Ann Richards was eighteen, a student with no history of psychiatric or any other serious illness, when she started taking oral contraceptives. Over a period of a year she became increasingly depressed, liable to burst into tears at any time and less and less able to cope. She suffered from unpredictable vomiting and daily bouts of uncontrollable crying. She was referred to a psychiatrist, and after a suicide attempt stayed in the university hospital until she was stabilised on antidepressants. She was treated with antidepressants (amitriptyline) and tranquillizers (chlordiazepoxide) for nine months, and the depression lifted a little. Returning to her course without the drugs she found it difficult to cope and suffered frequent migraine headaches. Nobody thought to question the role of her oral contraceptives in this dramatic change. Eventually she began to wonder if they might be part of the problem and ceased taking them. In the course of a week, she recalls, 'the whole world changed', she felt quite different and rapidly became her old self again. She was never seriously depressed again, although on two later attempts to take lower dose forms of the Pill the psychiatric reaction developed very quickly and depression and delusions forced her to give it up within weeks.

Among the most horrifying and extreme adverse reactions to drugs are teratogenesis, mutagenesis and carcinogenesis. Teratogenesis literally means the production of monsters. Thalidomide is a teratogen, though 'monster' is an insulting description of the victims, some of whom display more human and humane qualities than many of their more fortunate fellows. It is an unfortunate name for a disastrous process which can be initiated when drugs are taken during pregnancy. The timing can be crucial; thalidomide produces deformities only if it is taken between the third and eighth week, but if a woman takes a single dose on the fortieth day of her pregnancy, 'she can almost be given a written guarantee that her baby will be deformed'.[22] Thalidomide showed how widespread such a disaster could become; something like 8,000 thalidomide children survived in forty-six countries where the drug had been prescribed or sold over the counter to expectant mothers.[23]

Thalidomide is not typical of teratogens. Most are less predictable and consequently more elusive, because they will cause deformities in only a small proportion of the babies exposed to them while in the womb. The teratogenic properties of such drugs only emerge through careful statistical studies of huge populations. Even then sufficient uncertainty will remain to allow some experts to deny that drugs have the effect of damaging the unborn baby. In one study which assessed the role of drugs in causing congenital malformations, it was found that mothers of malformed babies were about 50 per cent more likely than mothers of normal babies to have taken one or more of the following drugs: progestogens to maintain pregnancy, tranquillizers or antibiotics. Nevertheless the authors felt able to conclude that these drugs were *not* teratogenic.[24]

Mutagenesis is damage to genetic material causing a permanent change in the characteristics that children will inherit from parents who have been damaged. Drug-induced changes in genetic material can cause defects that are passed on for generations, though the effects may not appear for many years. There is no totally adequate method of testing for mutagenesis, nor is it possible to know how many birth defects or childhood cancers may be caused by mutagenic drugs.

Carcinogenesis is the induction of cancer by any substance. Paradoxically, the most carcinogenic drugs are those used to treat cancers by causing chaotic disruption at the cellular level. Carcinogenic drugs also tend to be teratogenic and mutagenic.[25] There may be considerable delay between exposure to the drug and the appearance of disease, so it is frequently impossible to draw definite conclusions about cause and effect. Recent evidence suggests that reserpine (Serpasil), once widely used to control high blood pressure, causes breast cancer.[26] However, such suspicions are notoriously hard to verify.

It may be felt that in the above descriptions of the way drugs work and the possible adverse reactions they can produce, we have over-illuminated very rare occurrences, and that the vast majority of everyday drugs are perfectly safe. Unfortunately this is not true. Illness or death is part of the risk of any pharmacological intervention, much as injury and death are inevitable consequences of the mass use of motor vehicles.

At worst, iatrogenic disease can lead to premature and unnecessary death. At best, it will be one of the minor drug side-effects described earlier such as skin rash or drowsiness. As with road accidents, iatrogenesis involves a large element of chance and produces many thousands of minor ailments and inconveniences for every death. Between the extremes are the numbers of people who are unfortunately maimed and damaged in ways that can be permanent, and sometimes progressive.

Unlike road accidents, drug-induced diseases frequently present problems of recognition. People tend to become infirm towards the end of their lives, and this usually means that in the absence of any other treatment the rate of medication rises, with its attendant risks of drug interaction and increased adverse reaction rates.

Under these circumstances, the emergence of iatrogenic disease can be indistinguishable from a process of physical degeneration that might have occurred naturally. Diuretic drugs given for hypertension, for instance, can cause gout and diabetes in susceptible people,[27] but proof that the diuretic precipitated the disease relies on two pieces of evidence that are rarely available. The first is that withdrawal of the drug should lead to remission of symptoms, and the second that re-administration of the drug ('challenge') should cause them to return. Unfortunately some adverse reactions to drugs persist after their use has ceased. In these cases only those symptoms which are unique to iatrogenesis can be incontrovertibly attributed to the drug. It is therefore unusual for anyone to be told that he is suffering from drug-induced disease.

The euphoric assumptions underlying reliance on drug therapy inevitably lead to failure to recognise iatrogenesis as a major cause of disease, injury and death. There is a failure, also, to appreciate the depth to which assumptions about the value of drug therapy have penetrated the institutions surrounding health care.

The medical industry continues to behave as if its assumptions were correct, while objective examination of three assumptions is discouraged, and even suppressed.

Doctors often do not recognise the harm that their treatments may be causing. Even when there is a major and widely reported drug disaster with clear-cut features, a frighteningly high proportion of doctors do not seem to make the association. Relinquishment of hazardous drugs has been shown repeatedly to be disturbingly slow.[28] [29]

For the politicians who have the problem of providing, financing and controlling health care, drugs seem to offer an easy solution. With the structure of health care in the Western world, there is no easy way for politicians to balance demands against resources. And since there is almost always a short-term view, the line of greatest expediency is followed. Hospitals are being closed for lack of money to staff or run them while, ironically, resources trickle away with increasing speed from the pens of prescribing doctors. The long-term needs of health require provisions that go beyond a four- or five-year vote period and are therefore not attractive to most politicians, who prefer a demonstrable 'advance' within their period of office. A vicious circle is created: while resources are used illogically, the easiest and cheapest way to deal with the growing demand on health care is with drugs; but while more money is spent on drugs, less is available for other areas. It is a habit-forming philosophy with a momentum of its own.

Paul Ehrlich gave us the introduction to the underlying rationale of modern drug therapy. He concluded his insight into the possible dangers of chemicals as therapeutic agents by saying:

Magic substances like antibodies, which affect exclusively the harmful agent, will not be so easily found in the series of the artificially produced chemical substances. It must be regarded as in the highest degree probable that substances of this kind, foreign to the body, will be attracted also by the organs, and that, since we shall be dealing with a range of different substances, all with pronounced activities, these are not unlikely to injure the organism as a whole, or some part of it.[30]

It is regrettable that more attention was not paid to his doubts. The seductive simplicity of his initial idea has been pursued so enthusiastically that it has led to the availability of a range of around 28,000 substances 'with pronounced activities'. The injury they inflict has extended to the social, political and economic organism, as well as to a large number of individuals.

Chapter Three

Qualified Success

An often used quotation in books about drugs is a comment made in an address before the Massachusetts Medical Society in 1860 by Dr Oliver Wendell Holmes. He said: 'If the whole materia medica, as now used, could be sunk to the bottom of the sea, it would be better for mankind and all the worse for the fishes.'[1]

In 1860, the spectacular life-saving potential of the drugs upon which the reputation of pharmaceuticals has been built had not been realised. Would Holmes say the same today?

For this chapter we have selected some outstanding drug success stories. Most come from the small group of drugs which indisputably save life by treating conditions for which no other solution is known. These drugs are also characterised by offering great benefit with minimal risk, and their success gives a model of the power for good that pharmacology can offer; however as we shall see it is not success without qualification.

An early drug success was the development of vaccination against smallpox. Smallpox now exists only in medical and warfare research laboratories. A programme of world-wide vaccination coordinated by the World Health Organisation has ensured that even the most inaccessible and intractable reservoirs of the disease in India and Africa have been eradicated. To achieve this it was necessary for over 80 per cent of affected populations to be vaccinated or re-vaccinated within a five-year period.[2] The determination and resources required to overcome the logistic and technical problems involved were deployed with certainty of the success of a strategy that drew upon nearly two hundred years of successful immunisation.

Historically, attempts at crude immunisation against smallpox can be traced to the ancient Chinese and Arabs who would seek infection by a mild form of the disease in the belief that survival would confer immunity from a more virulent attack. Inoculation using pus from a person infected with a mild variant of smallpox was introduced to Western Europe by Lady Mary Wortley Montagu, wife of the British Ambassador to Constantinople. After careful testing on convicts and orphan children, the practice was adopted by the Hanoverian Kings of England, though there was some doubt and opposition from the Church.[3] Presumably, because God had given the disease to one person, it was interfering with divine purpose to transfer it to others.

Inoculation by this means was a risky procedure but smallpox was a dreaded disease. Even if it did not kill, it left its victims hideously scarred. About nine per cent of deaths in London between 1731 and 1765 were attributed to smallpox, and it had been recognised as a major threat in Europe since the fifteenth century. Spaniards had carried it with them to Mexico in 1520, and it eventually caused around three million Indian deaths and contributed substantially to the fall of the Aztec empire.

About 30 per cent of those infected died although epidemics varied, as did their effect on different populations. The usual method of transmission of the disease is by droplets of moisture in respiratory discharge, but material contaminated by lesions or their crusts can also be sources of infection. This fact was used by white settlers to introduce the disease deliberately to some North American Indian tribes by gifts of blankets contaminated with smallpox. Among these peoples the death rate was sometimes as high as 80 per cent.[4]

Edward Jenner, a country doctor in Gloucestershire, England, investigated the 'old wives' tale' that milkmaids who had suffered cow-pox, a mild disease carried by cows, did not get smallpox. In the late 1700s, a more cavalier medical ethic prevailed than that of today, and Jenner tried to inoculate with smallpox some people he had observed to be immune during local outbreaks. They failed to show symptoms of the disease. In 1796, Jenner performed his first successful immunisation, using cow-pox from a lesion on a milkmaid. He published his findings in 1798 and the procedure quickly replaced inoculation, giving a new word to the language: vaccination, from *Vacca*, Latin for cow.

Despite the widespread use of the vaccine, 85,900 cases of smallpox were recorded in the American continent between 1948 and 1952, with over 14,200 deaths.[5] The disease was sufficiently familiar for it to feature in a Laurel and Hardy film where the pair were quarantined in lodgings with their dog Laughing Gravy. In Africa and Asia the death rate remained high into the 1960s.

But by 1979, the World Health Organisation was able to announce that no new cases of the disease had been notified anywhere in the world.

Smallpox had been conquered with a freeze-dried form of Jenner's vaccine.

After Jenner's empirical success, the world had to wait over half a century, until the time of the American Civil War, for Louis Pasteur to provide the theoretical proof which became a significant component of modern medical practice. Pasteur was essentially a chemist and a veterinarian; he had no medical qualifications and his work was limited almost entirely to animals. However, he proved the germ theory of infection and transmittable disease to be correct, and was responsible for the revolution in thought that made us aware of the microsphere of life in many of its forms. From this awareness arose the realisation that rational action could be taken against diseases caused by micro-organisms. The theory of spontaneous generation, which had been held to be the cause of disease, was finally abandoned.

Pasteur's work led to the initiation of many modern practices, the use of antiseptics, aseptic surgery, bacteriology, epidemiology, immunisation in medicine, and various public health measures. His discovery of yeasts led to the process of pasteurisation and food preservation by canning.[6]

Through a happy accident with a culture of chicken cholera, Pasteur discovered that it was possible to attenuate bacteria and to produce vaccine in quantity. Attenuation allows live but non-virulent bacteria to be used in vaccines which are then capable of giving nearly total protection. He repeated the process with anthrax, demonstrating his mastery of the disease by a public display in June 1881, when twenty-five sheep, six oxen and an odd goat were vaccinated in public. A few days later they were equally publicly inoculated with virulent anthrax bacteria along with another twenty-five sheep, four cows and a second goat, none of which had been given the protective vaccination. After another few days, yet another public gathering of doctors, vets, scientists, farmers, administrators and peasants saw that all the unprotected animals were dead or dying of anthrax, whilst all those that had been vaccinated were healthy.

Pasteur's final triumph before his death in 1895 was to discover the means to protect people who had been bitten by a rabid animal, provided they reached him quickly enough. There are records of children being sent by boat and train to Paris from the United States, and of Russian peasants who had been ravaged by a mad wolf trekking to Paris with just one word of French: 'Pasteur'. Later the Csar was to become one of the largest subscribers to the foundation of the Institut Pasteur.[7]

The success of Pasteur's work in countering infectious organisms within the body set the course that anti-infective medicine would follow for seventy years. Its key was immunology, which concentrated on stimulating the body's own defence mechanisms to defeat invaders. Until the arrival of the sulphonamides and penicillin, this was the only way of coping with established infection. It is a line of medical endeavour which is still beneficially pursued today. In the 1960s, vaccines against measles and German measles (rubella) were developed; and in 1981 the Institut Pasteur Production received marketing approval for a hepatitis B vaccine, the first in the world.[8]

Despite its spectacular success, vaccination is only marginally helpful against rapidly adapting forms of infection such as influenza and the common cold. It also carries some risk. Usually the risk/benefit ratio is so low as to justify vaccination as a compulsory procedure among many populations, but with some diseases the benefits are not clear-cut. Controversy surrounds the use of whooping cough (pertussis) vaccine, particularly since social and environmental improvements had led to a dramatic decline in the severity and incidence of the disease *before* specific medical measures had been introduced to combat it. This decline was not accelerated by vaccination.[9] [10] Professor Gordon Stewart of Glasgow University has shown that vaccine damage is widespread, and that the protection conferred by the vaccine is slight. Vaccinated children are as likely to catch and transmit whooping cough as the un-vaccinated, though their symptoms may be less severe.[11] Nevertheless the British government continues to recommend that children be routinely vaccinated.

According to Professor Stewart, adverse reactions to whooping cough vaccination can often be predicted but the warnings are ignored. In a group of vaccine-damaged children, 65 per cent showed contra-indications to vaccination before the first injection. A further 20 per cent reacted adversely to their first exposure to the pertussis vaccine although they had shown no initial contra-indications, and they were given a second dose despite their reaction to the first. Further, 95 per cent of children who reacted adversely to one injection had similar or more severe reactions to subsequent exposures. Even so, 25 out of 143 children received three injections, reacting adversely to each.[12]

In all but a few of the children in Stewart's study, the adverse reaction was followed by arrest or loss of mental development and physical handicap ranging from spasticity to complete paralysis of all but the vital reflexes. Up to April 1981 the British Department of Health and Social Security had received 2,081 claims for damage to children due to pertussis vaccine, and 525 claims associated with other vaccines.[13] About a quarter of these had been accepted for awards under the Vaccine Damage Payments Act of 1979.[14]

In spite of its limitations, immunisation against infectious diseases must be regarded as a general good. The procedure, like other significant medical breakthroughs, suffers not so much from its own limitations as from the limitations of outlook it imposes on its practitioners. Too often a breakthrough in one area leads to a professional philosophy that tends towards the exclusion of other possibilities. The more significant the breakthrough, the more simplistic and ardent is the adherence of its advocates. This is not to say that they are necessarily wrong; but life has frequently shown itself to be unamenable to rigidly simplistic views.

In 1898 Sir Almroth Wright, then Professor of Pathology at the Army School of Medicine, developed a typhoid fever vaccine which was successfully demonstrated in India. At the outbreak of the Boer War, Wright wanted to have all British troops vaccinated before they left for active service; but the military medical establishment of the day would not hear of it. Consequently, typhoid took its traditional high toll of life in the war, and Wright resigned from the Army Medical School. He joined St Mary's Hospital in London and in 1908 became the founder and director of the Inoculation Department of the hospital. It was under Wright in this department that Sir Alexander Fleming spent most of his working life, and here that he did the work that led to his discovery of the antibiotic properties of penicillin.

Wright was absolutely convinced that doctors of the future would be immunologists, almost to the exclusion of any other discipline. His doctrine, 'Mobilise the Immunological Garrison', dominated the work of his department at St Mary's, which was at that time one of the most advanced centres of medical research in Britain. Although the Edinburgh surgeon Joseph Lister, following Pasteur's lead, had established carbolic acid as the standard antiseptic for preventing surgical wounds from *becoming* infected, few people believed that any substance would be found that could combat infection once it had entered the body, unless it were a vaccine.

This view was reinforced by work carried out at Boulogne on injured soldiers during the First World War. Fleming discovered that the use of antiseptics on infected open wounds reduced his patients' chances because the antiseptic killed more phagocytes, the white blood cells which ingest bacteria, than infecting organisms.[15]

Antiseptics were not 'magic bullets'. Some parts of the chemical industry, notably those in Germany, had not, however, given up the search for Ehrlich's selective antagonist. During the first quarter of this century many new ranges of antiseptics were developed and marketed, and naturally great claims were made for each new product; but each was equally useless against germs inside the body.

Indeed the proliferation of these substances led Professor Ronald Hare, then working on puerperal fever at Queen Charlotte's Maternity Hospital in London, to complain in exasperation of 'another of those damned compounds from Germany with a trade name and of unknown composition that are no use anyway'. Hare later explained: 'What I thought on this occasion may bring home to those who did not live through this period what bacteriologists thought about chemical compounds for the treatment of bacteriological infections. None of us, not even the inhabitants of the

Inoculation Department, were hostile to them. But we were, time and again, infuriated by the claims put forward by clinicians and commercial firms for compounds that should never have been introduced into medicine at all.'[16]

These background attitudes contributed to the delay in the recognition and development of penicillin after Fleming noticed its effect on his culture plates. It is necessary to examine briefly an earlier chemotherapeutic success to see how the necessary change in outlook occurred.

This success was the first of the sulpha drugs. It was announced by Dr Gerhard Domagk, director of research in the German company Bayer. His paper, published in February 1935, reported on work he had carried out in 1932 with Prontosil, a dyestuff that had displayed remarkable antibacterial properties. Among these was the fact that, unlike antiseptics, it did not kill both bacteria and body cells indiscriminately.

In his exhaustive research, Domagk had shown that Prontosil was inactive against bacteria in a test tube, but was active and effective in living animals. This apparent anomaly was explained by a French husband-and-wife team working at the Institut Pasteur, Dr Jacques and Mme Trefouel, who showed that the chemical was broken down within the body and that it was the sulphanilamide component that attacked the bacteria. Their analysis was confirmed in 1936 by Dr Albert Fuller who had demonstrated that patients being treated with Prontosil excreted sulphanilamide in their urine.

Sulphanilamide did not unleash the commercial endeavour that was later to surround penicillin, possibly because its discovery had been noted in 1908 and it could not therefore be protected by patent in Germany. It did however, provide the sort of dramatic cameo that cinema audiences have come to expect of medical dramas: Dr Domagk's daughter Hildegarde was knitting one day when she pricked her finger with a needle. She developed septicaemia and her father used his newly discovered drug to cure her.

After the excitement of the initial discovery, sulphanilamide was found to be useful only against a limited group of infections. Its action relies on interference with the life-cycle of a bacterium by a process which involves stealing the enzymes the bacteria need for their development; but this is only effective with certain types of bacteria. Nevertheless it caused a marked conceptual shift. At one level it prompted chemical and pharmaceutical companies to set up their own research departments to seek further sulpha-type drugs. ICI took this action in 1936.

At a more profound level, it caused the medical establishment to reconsider its attitudes to the possibility of chemotherapy. Professor Hare put it thus: 'The fact remains that his [Domagk's] was one of the most important medical discoveries that has ever been made, for it not only enables us to treat and cure a whole series of very serious forms of infection, but of even greater importance, it showed us how wrong had been our ideas about how a successful chemotherapeutic agent was likely to act. As a consequence of this, penicillin began to be thought of as a possible alternative. But let there be no doubt about it, without the sulphonamides to show the way, it is improbable that penicillin would have emerged from its obscurity.'[17]

Penicillin is produced by *Penicillium* moulds. Its medicinal history begins in Italy with Dr B. Gosio in 1896. He was investigating cases of pellagra, a vitamin deficiency disease, among agricultural workers in northern Italy. In the course of this work he found fifteen different organisms infecting the corn they ate, one of which was *Penicillium glaucum*, which Gosio cultured in a variety of different liquids, some similar to those used in penicillin cultures today. Gosio found that his culture would stop the growth of anthrax germs in a test tube; but he lacked the resources and perspective to pursue this discovery.

Alexander Fleming noticed in 1928 that mould growing on one of his staphylococcal culture plates had destroyed the surrounding colonies of bacteria. He went on to isolate the mould and found that the fluid beneath it had anti-bacterial properties. More importantly, he discovered that it displayed a remarkable lack of toxicity. Even when fluid equal to 25 per cent of a mouse's body weight was injected into the animal it showed no toxic effects.

Fleming continued to work on penicillin and its purification until 1937. His rate of progress must be viewed in the context of medical research at that time: it was predominantly carried out by doctors who depended on their fee-paying patients to make a living. Their research brought little, if any, income. Most research centres such as that at St Mary's also manufactured their own vaccines and sera, which the doctors then used. In those days there was no industrial involvement in medicine as we have come to know it.

At Oxford, Florey, Chain and Heatley began extracting and purifying penicillin from mould cultures. The difficulty of this process meant that enormous quantities of culture brew were required, about 100 litres (over 20 gallons) for one day's treatment. By February 1941 there was enough penicillin to attempt the treatment of an Oxford policeman who was dying of staphylococcal pyraemia. The infection was arrested and the patient rallied. But the penicillin supply ran out and he died.

As with so many discoveries, penicillin had to be taken out of Britain before it could be produced in a way that would fulfil its promise. In 1941, Florey and Heatley took it to the United States, where government, industry and universities cooperated to make sufficient funds and facilities available. By 1943, under the sponsorship of the War Production Board,

American enterprise was unleashed on penicillin, and a boom followed. There is even record of a backyard operation producing batches of penicillin in old whisky bottles in Brooklyn. By 1946, penicillin production was at a high enough level for the drug to be released for use among civilian populations.

The enduring reputation of penicillin was earned both by its near miraculous anti-bacterial properties and by its safety. It is an extraordinary fact that the first true antibiotic to be discovered should not only be the most useful and the least toxic, but that it should remain so after many others have been discovered or manufactured. The reason for this lies in the way penicillin works.

Unlike mammalian cells, bacterial cells have thick walls upon which the integrity of the organisms depend. If the wall is breached the cell bursts and the organism dies. Some spherical bacteria, such as the streptococci which cause wound infections, septicaemia, scarlet fever and severe bacterial sore throat, can withstand pressures equal to twenty atmospheres.[18] The remarkable strength depends on the cross-linked structure of the cell wall, which is formed essentially from large molecules of muramic and teichoic acid. The penicillin molecule incorporates itself into the building process and causes catastrophic disruption. The drug is so basically safe because neither muramic nor teichoic acid are found in human cells.

Because of the way penicillin works, it is essential that enough is used for sufficient time to ensure that each individual bacterium is killed at its appropriate stage of post-reproductive growth. Failure in this respect encourages survivors to adapt their chemistry and become resistant. Ironically those strains of bacteria which are resistant produce a substance called penicillinase which in turn disrupts the penicillin molecule by splitting the essential side-chains from the nucleus and rendering it inactive.[19]

Penicillin G, the original form discovered by Fleming, is still the antibiotic of choice for some serious infections such as bacterial endocarditis (inflammation of the lining of the heart and its valves), which was previously incurable. The treatment of many infections was revolutionised by penicillin; the venereal diseases syphilis and gonorrhoea are readily treated, often with a single dose, though certain strains of gonorrhoea are now becoming resistant. Lobar pneumonia, which used to strike healthy people without warning and produced a mortality rate of about 30 per cent in the 1930s, has been conquered. The anxious wait of up to ten days for the 'crisis' when the patient's fever dropped dramatically with the victory of his immune responses has been cut to a mere day or so with a negligible risk.[20]

As with other drugs with a profound effect, the impact of penicillin was not limited to the sphere of medicine. The vast commercial possibilities of drugs were finally appreciated, and virtually every United States pharmaceutical company launched a massive programme of screening soils, dusts and moulds from every part of the world, searching for more useful fungi.

Further antibiotics followed. In 1944, Professor Waksman of Rutgers University, working as a consultant to Merck, announced the discovery of streptomycin, the first broad-spectrum antibiotic. The year 1947 saw Parke Davis & Co. announcing chloramphenicol, a molecule they were able to synthesise by 1949 to produce the first synthetic antibiotic. Aureomycin was produced by Lederle Laboratories in 1948, and Terramycin by Pfizer in 1950.[21] Progress on the antibiotic trail is followed in further detail elsewhere in this book.

Each antibiotic is capable of making a valuable contribution to human welfare, provided it is correctly used and not treated as a universal medicament. Pencillin particularly has suffered from overuse and misuse. Its lack of toxicity has encouraged casual prescribing, with the result that more and more strains of resistant bacteria have emerged. The chances of encountering penicillin resistance in infections acquired in hospital are very high. When penicillin was first introduced, almost all staphylococcal infections (such as abcesses) responded favourably. Now about 90 per cent of staphylococcal infections acquired in hospital are resistant. Outside hospitals around 20 per cent are found to have acquired similar resistance.[22]

The second most spectacular drug discovery of this century is probably that of insulin by Banting and Best at McGill University in 1921. Most juvenile-onset diabetics depend on insulin for their day-to-day survival. Sir Derrick Dunlop, one-time president of the British Committee on Safety of Medicines, wrote: 'It is doubtful if there has ever been a medical discovery comparable in drama to the effect of the administration of these precious vials of insulin. . . . Patients did recover from severe infections, even septicaemias, without the use of drugs, but those emaciated acute diabetics living on their impossibly high-fat, low-carbohydrate diets, surrounded by an aura of acetone, were invariably doomed to rapid extinction.'[23]

Diabetes mellitus is a metabolic disorder characterised by an excessively high blood-sugar level. It has been estimated that there are 200 million diabetics in the world.[24] Not all depend on insulin; in the United States, probably half of those diagnosed as diabetic could be free of the disease if they were willing to reduce weight so dramatically that instead of being obese they were lean. For these mature-onset diabetics, the disease is almost invariably a consequence of overweight and excessive sugar consumption. It is avoidable and can usually be cured without the use of drugs. Predictably, since this cure would involve sacrifice on the part of the patient and some possible loss of income and power for the doctor, the majority of overweight diabetics are treated with oral anti-diabetic drugs[25] that involve hazards that we describe elsewhere.

Unlike overweight mature-onset diabetics, those who develop the disease under the age of twenty or so cannot choose to cure themselves. Whereas mature diabetics often produce normal amounts of natural insulin which they are unable to utilise, in people who become diabetic as juveniles, insulin production declines dramatically, approaching and in many cases reaching zero. This results in severe metabolic aberrations. Body protein is lost in the urine and carbohydrate and fat metabolism is disrupted. Toxic acid (ketone) substances accumulate in the body, the patient loses weight very fast, and suffers from nausea, vomiting, excessive urination, thirst and often hunger. Without insulin the patient becomes very weak and eventually loses consciousness and dies. Starvation was the only treatment before insulin; it might extend the patient's life to three or even four years from the onset of the disease.

In 1909, de Mayer gave the name 'insulin' to a substance secreted by the pancreas, a large gland lying near the stomach. Banting and Best gave a diabetic dog pancreatic extract and isolated reasonably pure insulin in 1921. Only recently has insulin been synthesised, and diabetics generally use insulin derived from pigs or cattle. It is destroyed by digestive jucies and has to be taken by injection: an unpleasant chore, but, as Dr Lawrence, the first British diabetic to use Banting and Best's new discovery commented, 'People who have been very ill and wasted and nearly dead would have had a hundred injections a day if it had made them feel as well as it did.'[26]

Even with injections of insulin, the diabetic's life is far from normal. Dr Lawrence wrote in 1925, 'I would point out to diabetics and their friends that they owe their lives to medical research'; and indeed they do; but their lives are still, on average, only half the normal length. Dr E.P. Joslin, an expert on diabetes, kept records of his patients' progress from 1897, when he started in practice. From 1897 to 1914, the average duration of diabetes (of all kinds) at death was 4.9 years; 19.4 per cent of diabetics died within one year, 67 per cent in less than five years. By 1957 the average duration of the disease was 18.2 years, with only 1.6 per cent of patients dying within one year and 9 per cent in less than five years.[27]

Because it replaces an essential naturally occurring secretion, insulin is virtually free of adverse effects. Some diabetics are allergic to cow or pig insulin because it is slightly different from the protein their own bodies would produce. Is insulin, then, an exception to the general rule that potent drugs can be dangerous?

Unfortunately, medical practice can make even such a benign substance as insulin into a dangerous drug. Over-use of insulin is something the diabetic learns to avoid very quickly because it causes a severe fall in blood sugar which can develop into serious hypoglycaemia and finally, if it is unchecked by food intake, the patient can lapse into a hypoglycaemic coma, a condition which can cause brain damage if it persists or is indulged in too frequently.

Insulin coma 'therapy' was used on many non-diabetic psychiatric patients before being replaced by the more easily managed electro-convulsive therapy (ECT). This misuse of insulin was pioneered by Manfred Sakel in Vienna in the doubly misguided belief that the hypo-thalamus was the seat of psychoses and that he could alter its function with insulin. His work began with the use of insulin as a sedative in the treatment of morphine withdrawal. When some patients suffered con-vulsions, he added barbiturates. Then he tried it on patients suffering from mental illness, and in 1933 he reported on the beneficial effects of repeated insulin coma. Sakel used this treatment, particularly on schizo-phrenics, from 1936 until his death in New York in 1957.

During the 1940s, insulin coma and subcoma were considered important forms of treatment for schizophrenia. The unfortunate patients were easier to manage after they had been subjected to up to fifty episodes of hypo-glycaemic coma daily induced by large doses of extra insulin. The seizures that occurred were not considered to be part of the therapeutic process.[28]

Pernicious anaemia is another disease that was invariably fatal. It is a symptom of vitamin B_{12} deficiency. The development of red blood cells is arrested, so that too few are formed, and those are frequently misshapen and fragile. Lasck of vitamin B_{12} also affects the nervous system and can cause partial paralysis of the limbs.

Very few diets are deficient in natural vitamin B_{12}. Problems are nearly always due to the body's failure to absorb the vitamin. Pernicious anaemia was first described in 1849, but it was not until 1926 that Minot and Murphy showed that it could be treated by feeding sufferers with raw liver. Vitamin B_{12} was found to be the curative factor (it is stored in the liver) and isolated in 1948; its chemical structure was established in 1955. The disease is now treated with regular injections of the vitamin, and sufferers can live completely normal lives.[29]

Vitamin B_{12} is unique in that it is practically specific for one well-defined condition whose prevalence is known; it is only of use in treating pernicious anaemia. Because of this, it was selected for an epidemiological study by Cochrane and Moore.[30] They found that more than three times as much vitamin was prescribed as was reasonably calculated to be required, even given that doctors might use an unnecessarily high dose for each sufferer. In Denmark, when oral forms of B_{12} were added to injectable forms and compared with ideal quantities required, the excessive con-sumption was found to cost twenty times as much as the total calculated to be necessary.

Fortunately, vitamin B_{12} is not a dangerous drug. Overdosage at the level discovered by Cochrane and Moore would not cause direct damage to the patients involved. It merely provides a better than usual example of documented over-prescribing and misuse of resources.

The replacement of a vital bodily substance such as insulin or vitamin B_{12}, where the body cannot be stimulated to rectify the deficiency, is obviously a safe and desirable use of drug technology. It enables normal life processes to continue. There are, however, times when it may be more desirable to suppress or inhibit normal bodily reactions. In this area, one type of drug has revolutionised the possibilities of medical intervention: the anaesthetic.

Surgery no longer inspires the terror of the past. Through the use of anaesthesia, sophisticated procedures that could not have been considered a century or more ago have become routine. Introducing a collection of papers on anaesthesia, Cole[31] wrote:

> Surgery means pain. It consists of cutting, pulling, and sewing; it includes 'manipulating' joints, sawing bones, and slicing skin. It is made up of all the separate maneuvers that have been actually used as forms of torture. Without anaesthesia surgery must be hurried, is necessarily limited to minor procedures or is needlessly destructive, can only be palliative, and is synonymous with pain.

Anaesthesia has evolved steadily since 1800, when Humphrey Davy published the results of a study of nitrous oxide which showed the possibility of its use as an anaesthetic. He suggested that it might be used for operations, but nobody took any notice of this for over forty years. Later when Wells attempted to demonstrate nitrous oxide anaesthesia in Boston in 1844 he failed, and another twenty years was to elapse before it was successfully used.

The year 1846 was the turning point when anaesthesia was used in both Britain and America. Morton used ether successfully for tooth extraction and for surgery. The discovery was taken up fast, and within a few months ether had revolutionised surgery and had been used for labour pains. In 1847 Simpson used chloroform for surgery, finding it easier to use than ether. There was controversy concerning the relative merits of the two drugs for the next fifty years, until ether was proved safer.

The next group of anaesthetic drugs was developed in the 1920s. These included ethylene and cyclopropane. The discovery of hexobarbitone, a rapidly metabolised injectible anaesthetic, led in 1932 to the successful clinical use of intravenous anaesthesia. The volatile inhaled anaesthetics had a small margin of safety because the concentration necessary to produce light anaesthesia is about half that which paralyses the respiratory centre. Increased practical safety was achieved through the use of pre-medication, which reduced the quantity of anaesthetic required.[32]

Anaesthesia had vociferous opponents. There were religious objections, especially to its use in childbirth, where it was argued that anaesthesia was immoral because it interfered with God's will that women should suffer. In 1853, the *Lancet* stamped firmly on the rumour that Queen Victoria had been given chloroform at the birth of her seventh child, pronouncing the very idea irresponsible. For Her Majesty's part, she wrote in her diary of 'that blessed chloroform'. Simpson went so far as to publish a pamphlet defending anaesthesia on the basis that Adam's rib had been removed 'while our primogenitor was in a state of stupor', thus if God could do it, surely he would not object if man did likewise. Predictably, the editor of the *Lancet* disagreed.[33]

There were of course some deaths as techniques evolved. Fischer, who developed barbiturate anaesthesia, was the first to take his own life with barbiturates. He had family troubles and cancer.[34]

Today, although some patients suffer such adverse effects as halothane-induced jaundice, the hazards of anaesthesia are mainly indirect. They permit unnecessary and potentially risky surgery which would not otherwise be considered. One example is that the rate of hysterectomy in the United States has been shown to depend directly upon the number of surgeons working in a given area. Therapeutically unjustifiable operations, such as coronary bypass surgery, would not be possible without sophisticated anaesthetic techniques.

In more modern times one of the major strategies employed by the pharmacologists and biochemists in their search for new drugs is to isolate chemicals involved in disease processes, and to look for others which will produce a particular desirable effect on them. Sir Henry Dale, who worked at the Wellcome Research Laboratories in the early years of this century, was a pioneer of this technique.

Dale's research on ergot, a poisonous fungus which grows on rye, led him to the discovery of histamine and acetylcholine, and prepared the way for further innovation in pharmacology. Acetylcholine is now recognised as one of a group of neurotransmitters. Electrical impulses travel along nerves and cause the release of the contents of millions of tiny containers of neurotransmitting chemicals at the ends of the nerve. Acetylcholine conveys information in this way from nerve endings to muscle fibres and stimulates the muscle to contract. The acetylcholine molecule does this specifically by locking onto a compatible molecule at the receptor site, and drugs can be used to influence this action.

This knowledge has been put to valuable use with the development of beta-blocking drugs. Angina sufferers experience pain when the heart is stimulated by excitement or exercise; this is because the choked coronary arteries deliver too little oxygen-rich blood to supply the heart muscle. First, pharmacologists sought a method of increasing the oxygen supply to the heart. Failing in this, they searched for a means of limiting the action of the particular neurotransmitter which stimulates the heart muscle. ICI's success in discovering propranolol, a chemical which has this effect, led to the development of the group of beta-blockers, drugs which have become enormously popular and widely used. They are credited with saving the lives of many sufferers from hypertension and heart disease, and with making a great many angina patients comfortable.[35]

Timolol (Blocadren), Merck, Sharp & Dohme's beta-blocker, has been credited with preventing cardiac deaths in patients who have suffered a heart attack. A multi-centre study in Norway involving 1,884 heart attack patients showed a considerably reduced death-rate in the high-risk group, and some reduction in deaths among the lower-risk patients.[36] In Britain, the CSM has accepted this trial as evidence of the efficacy of timolol for the prevention of repeat heart attacks which often follow within a short period after the first.[37]

The results of a five year study of the effects of beta-blocker treatment of mild and moderate hypertensives[38] showed that these drugs do reduce both morbidity and mortality when compared with no treatment. The study involved 961 people, 382 of whom had normal blood pressure and acted as controls. Initially 392 were defined as hypertensive, and in this group blood pressure was reduced to normal with beta-blockers. For a third group, control of blood pressure was incomplete, and members had pressures above the criterion level on at least 20 per cent of occasions. Finally, seventy-six patients remained untreated. The results showed clearly that beta-blockade led to a marked reduction in ischaemic heart disease and cerebro-vascular disease. Better control of blood pressure produced better results.

The design of this study did not allow for any non-drug methods of treatment. The people involved were questioned about their smoking, dietary and exercise habits, but they were given no advice on the effects of these on their condition. So although it may demonstrate the advantages of beta-blockade over no treatment for hyptertensive patients, it does not compare drug with non-drug treatment. By contrast, penicillin proved its benefits not through comparison with untreated disease, but by its superiority to any treatment previously available.

With the changes that have taken place in the dominant types of disease it may be that therapeutic advance is inevitably less dramatic. Acute illness and death due to infection can be halted almost miraculously with antibiotic therapy. In these cases the disease process occurs in a previously relatively healthy body and there may be little, if any, structural damage. The same is not true of the heart disease patient. By the time he suffers his first attack, signs of cumulative damage to circulatory system are widespread. Years of misuse and neglect have led to his situation, and no magic bullet could possibly reverse it within a short period, if at all. The advantages of drug therapy for such conditions are therefore bound to be limited and equivocal.

It may be that we must now recognise that we are approaching the end of the medical legacy bequeathed by Pasteur. We now await the findings of progressive detailed exploration of the complex inter-molecular relationships between parts of our bodies, and of our protagonists. The situation is further complicated for medicine by the fact that today we are confronted with disease patterns that are multi-causal, and usually environmental. There seems little likelihood that drugs will provide long-term answers to these problems. And indeed the question might also be raised, is it desirable that we should expect them to do so?

Within this framework it is difficult to define requirements for an indisputably successful drug. Hundreds, indeed thousands, of the products of the pharmaceutical industry are effective for certain defined and limited indications. Others may be deemed effective according to the biases of some observers, but not so by others with different attitudes. The point is that the question is now social or political, rather than medical.

An obvious example of this is to be found in the enormously successful range of psychotropic drugs. There are those who argue that these products are virtually worthless because, by their nature, they are palliatives which leave fundamental problems unsolved. Few would take such a hard line view; after all, insulin cannot *cure* diabetes, but it is appropriately used to treat it. At the other extreme there are those who consider that it is quite reasonable to use potent tranquillisers to quieten prisoners, patients and populations alike.

Possibly cimetidine (Tagamet), a drug developed for ulcer patients, represents the closest approach to a recent dramatic success story. Often the only alternative is major surgery.

Stomach (gastric) and duodenal ulcers are caused by stress and poor dietary habits. In order to digest the food we eat, the stomach produces a substance called pepsinogen, which becomes the protein-digesting enzyme pepsin in the presence of hydrochloric acid which is secreted by cells in the stomach. This potent mixture is quite capable of digesting the stomach itself, but is generally prevented from doing so by the presence of food and a layer of mucous over the extra-tough cells of the stomach lining. Acid is normally only secreted when there is food to absorb it, but when stomach emptying is delayed the highly acid mixture of contents can begin to damage the lining. Normally the acid is neutralised by the alkaline environment of the duodenum, but again the food must move along efficiently for the process to work properly.

Emotional stress is a familiar cause of stomach upset. In animal experiments psychologists have discovered that ulcers develop quickly when animals are subjected to punishment which they cannot avoid, and which are unpredictable in timing and severity. In one particularly gruesome experiment rats were found to develop ulcers in as little as an hour and a half under these conditions.

Obviously few people are subjected to the sort of torture inflicted on animals by unimaginative psychologists. But the elements of unpredictability and uncontrollability are present in the lives of many people. For some, driving in heavy traffic might fulfil these criteria, for others it could be working for a hypercritical boss, or the continual pressure of business problems.

Dolphins develop ulcers when they are kept in captivity for our amusement. It was on these highly intelligent and playful animals that cimetidine was tested. Cimetidine suppresses substances which stimulate gastric secretion by selectively blocking histamine receptors. With the reduction in destructive stomach secretion the ulcers can begin to heal.[39]

Cimetidine is a new drug, only recently accepted for use in some parts of the world. In 1981 the Japanese drug regulatory body was still considering its use.[40] There are fears that it has serious adverse effects, that it possibly causes stomach cancer, although this is a difficult question because ulcers can be symptoms of cancer which the drug will then mask.[41] Over the six years up to January 1981 the British Committee on Safety of Medicines had received 2,459 reports of possible adverse reactions to cimetidine.[42]

On the other hand cimetidine has reduced the surgery rate in those countries where it is used. According to a survey published in the *Lancet*,[43] a sudden and drastic fall in the number of operations for duodenal ulcer followed the introduction of cimetidine. The reduction was most noticeable in 1976–7, coinciding with the introduction of the drug. Nationwide in Britain these operations are down by 40 per cent, and it seems that the extent of the reduction is closely correlated with the popularity of the drug; in some centres vigorous medical treatment with high doses of cimetidine has resulted in an 80 per cent reduction in elective surgery.[44]

Predictably, ulcers tend to return when medication is stopped. Cimetidine provides effective symptomatic relief for many ulcer sufferers, but it does nothing to treat the cause of the problem. Like so many recent pharmacological 'breakthroughs', cimetidine is effective if medication is continued indefinitely. Indefinite medication is all too likely to lead to problems with adverse reactions. Are these conditions that we are now content to accept to consider a drug as a success?

As with many other things in life the assessment of success has become more complex in recent times. Antibiotics and replacement therapies were dramatically and obviously successful because there was no other answer, and the results of their use were generally unambiguous. Drugs used as anaesthetics, or even as analgesics, are generally beneficial because they facilitate other curative processes, although these processes can themselves become the subject of abuse.

Increasingly it is the context in which a particular drug is used which determines whether it can be considered successful or not. This requires that drug use be considered against all the possible alternative therapies, and also that the social effects of widespread use be considered. To illustrate the latter point, it has been argued that starvation was a side-effect of the successful use of anti-malarial drugs in some parts of the world, because the drugs increased the survival rate of the populations in excess of available food supplies.[45] In those circumstances was the use of anti-malarial drugs a success or a failure? Or was it simply short-sighted and inappropriate to the real problems of the people involved?

As many drugs now shelter in the reflected glory of the few, their acceptance as beneficial substances depends increasingly upon our assumptions about them. It also becomes clear that only the passage of time and wider experience beyond the immediate medical tradition will lead us to a more realistic perspective that will enable accurate judgements to be made.

Chapter Four

The Medicine Men

The trouble is, they (the pharmaceutical industry) have so much money to spend.
– Bill Haddad, ex-aide to Senator Estes Kefauver
at the time of the Kefauver Hearings, speaking
during BBC Radio 4's 'In Sickness and in
Wealth', 3rd September 1979.

We trust the drug companies. They wouldn't lie to us.
– Dr Virginia Ramirez de Barquero, Department
of Drugs, Ministry of Health, Costa Rica. Quoted
in Silverman, M., *The Drugging of the Americas*,
Berkeley, University of California Press, 1976

The patent medicines business, together with the established pharmacy of time-tested substances, was the predecessor of the modern drug industry.[1] The first recorded patent medicine was probably 'Anderson's Pills', on sale in Britain during the reign of Elizabeth I (1558–1603). Through the seventeenth and eighteenth centuries large numbers of highly idiosyncratic remedies, such as Dr Bateman's Pectoral Drops, Daffy's Elixir and so on, became increasingly popular. Some of them worked, some did not. Their medicinal properties included a large element of luck.

The British enthusiasm spread across the Atlantic and these medicines became popular in America. In 1824, the Philadelphia College of Pharmacy published a pharmacopoeia which only listed the most popular British patent medicines. However, by 1850, the Americans had established their own range of patent specifics, like Widow Read's Ointment for the Itch, Dr Swaynes' Consumption Cure and Samuel Lee's Bilious Pills, and these were beginning to appear on the British market. It was a boom era for the patent-medicine men on both sides of the Atlantic and the manufacturers promoted their wares enthusiastically. One, Thomas Beecham, tried to have his pills advertised on the white cliffs of Dover.

There was a lot of money to be made. Among the early trail blazers was Joanna Stephens, who in 1738 sold her secret cure to the British nation for £5,000, not doing quite as well as Dr Goddard, who had pulled the same trick a century earlier with his formula for Goddard's Drops, for which secret the government parted with £6,000. The most enduring success was achieved by an Irish quack purveyor of patent medicines. John St John

Long. He made a fortune by selling an ointment which was said to be working if it caused irritation and discoloration. He sold it in great quantities from his premises in Harley Street, London.

Humble beginnings have resulted in major international ventures. The Plough Court Pharmacy opened for business in 1715, supplying the public and various London physicians. It has since metamorphosed into a major pharmaceutical company, Allen & Hanbury Ltd, and subsequently into a part of the multinational giant Glaxo. In 1816, H.E. Merck started work as an apothecary, making up bottles of medicine for sale. By 1822 he had set up as a wholesale distributor, and today the name lives on in E. Merck Ltd and Merck, Sharp & Dohme Ltd. Thomas Beecham began as a chemist in Wigan, Lancashire. In 1847 he founded a company to sell Beecham's Pills, and twenty years later had established his product in America. Beecham's stayed with 'patent', or over-the-counter, medicines until their entry into the ethical pharmaceutical market in 1949 on the post-war penicillin boom. It was a Beecham laboratory that first isolated the active penicillin nucleus, thus removing the last hurdle from the cheap mass-production of synthetic penicillins.

The Germans and the Swiss had become the leading industrial chemists in the latter part of the industrial revolution, and a large number of major drug manufacturers developed in these countries as offshoots of the chemical dyestuffs industry. Basle, in Switzerland, is a traditional textile centre, and dyestuffs manufacturers located themselves there to supply the needs of the textile processors. Three of the biggest drug companies in the world, founded towards the end of the nineteenth century to make dyes, still have plants near Basle: Ciba-Geigy, Sandoz and Hoffmann-La Roche.

Until Erhlich's discovery of Salvarsan in 1907, the dyestuffs industry regarded drug production as an incidental opportunity to get rid of waste by-products and make a little money in the process. Bucheim, a major pharmacologist who also taught the History of Medicine, is recorded as having complained in the mid nineteenth century that:

> The chemical industry of our days produces various substances for which no market can be found. Under these circumstances the idea suggests itself that it might be possible to use these products as drugs. We know that a great number of physicians, without rhyme or reason, go after every new remedy that is recommended to them. If any industrialist is but shrewd enough to advertise sufficiently he usually succeeds in increasing the sale of the product – for some time at least – and thus enriching himself.[2]

The success of this strategy for shrewd industrialists had to wait for equally shrewd men to play their part in others areas. Before William

Brockedon, a Devon artist, had trouble securing the graphite in his pencils, all pills were made by hand. This made mass marketing difficult. In 1843 Brockedon was granted patent number 9977 for a device for 'shaping Pills, Lozenges and Black lead by pressure in Dies'. Within a year *Pharmaceutical Journal* was able to report, 'We have received a specimen of bicarbonate of potash compressed into the form of a pill by a process invented by Mr Brockedon and for which he has taken out a patent. We understand the process is applicable to the compression of a variety of other substances into a solid mass, without the intervention of gum or other adhesive material'.[3] Their understanding was perfectly correct, and the hand-rolling of pills was added to the list of dying arts.

The *cachet*, or capsule, was invented by a French chemist in 1833. Although not as amenable to mass production as pills, or tablets as Burroughs Wellcome called them in 1878, they do have some practical advantages, as well as allowing opportunity for applications of colour art that may owe more to magic than necessity.

The last step in the development of suitable means of delivery of mass-produced drugs was taken in 1853 when the first hypodermic injection was given by Alexander Wood of Edinburgh. He injected morphine into an elderly spinster, using sherry as a solvent.

With these three inventions the way was clear for the production, distribution, and administration of drugs to mass markets. And so those companies which had successful products or successful promotion strategies grew and consolidated their positions.

Some pharmaceutical discoveries led to spectacular riches, and since the possibilities for innovation and development appeared as limitless as the market for the products, more and more people were encouraged to enter the business in search of the enormous profits which could be made.

There was competition and freedom at this stage of the development of pharmaceutical companies within various nations. But as the pressures of competition increased, the firms in all areas of chemical manufacturing found that their domestic markets were wholly inadequate for the size to which economic factors forced them to grow. Because of economies of scale, it can be as easy to produce one hundred tons of a drug as it is to produce one; and this, coupled with the growing need for large promotion and research programmes, forced the drug manufacturers to expand beyond their domestic boundaries and home markets.[4]

As with patent medicines, the obvious way to expand the market was by exporting the finished product. Drugs are light and easy to handle in relation to their value, so the additional transport costs were negligible. But expansion came to involve political issues, and the politicians' requirements gave birth to the multinational giants that now dominate the world pharmaceutical industry.

The First World War of 1914–18 provided the motivation for these political pressures. Many countries found that medicines they had taken for granted were produced by a country that was now an enemy. The British and United States governments, among others, have since that time fostered the growth of a home-based drug manufacturing industry. Governments encouraged domestic production and discouraged imports by the conventional means of high tariffs and direct trade controls, and production licences were more likely to be granted to those firms prepared to establish local manufacture behind the protective wall of prohibitive import restrictions.[5]

With this broad-brush encouragement, the growth of some drug manufacturers has been spectacular in the extreme. One analyst, writing in 1971, summarised the situation for Eli Lilly & Co. at the end of the golden decades of the 1950s and 1960s thus: 'The most rapid development accompanied by the greatest number of changing circumstances has taken place in the last few years. Eli Lilly & Co., for example, is 96 years old; yet in terms of growth, it took 75 years to reach the first $100 million sales level, 14 years to reach $200 million, 4 years to attain $300 million, and only 2 years for $400 million and a little more than a year for $500 million.'[6]

This picture of growth was reflected by other major companies, for although some 5,000 companies in Europe and America were making products for a £2,000 million drug market in the mid 1960s, around thirty multinational corporations had become dominant. In national order of might, the American and Swiss multinational drug companies are closely followed by German and British ones.

The interests of these giants, apart from pharmaceuticals, range from the predictable veterinary preparations, pesticides, herbicides and fertilisers, to paints, plastics, soft drinks, foods and food additives, toiletries and cosmetics. In fact, they cover most products which can be made by manipulation around the carbon molecule.

The primary concern of these Western multinationals is to make new artificial molecules and to find profitable uses for them. Natural products, the traditional components of drugs, are rarely desired. Herb gardens are peculiar to Japanese drug companies, one of which has a plantation with over four thousand different plants as part of its research and development section.[7] There is no parallel in the West.

The molecular manipulation approach is highly successful in business terms. A report of America's Pharmaceutical Manufacturers' Association noted that 'The US pharmaceutical manufacturers have 277 plants, 367 sales offices, and 554 distributors in various parts of the world. Of the plants, 39 per cent are located in Latin America and 29 per cent in Europe.'[8]

A more detailed picture of what this means on the ground can be achieved by looking at the countries where three US multinationals have established foreign subsidiaries.[9]

Estimated rank and turnover for the year ending June 1980
of the top multinational drug manufacturers

Rank	Multinational	Country	Sales ($ million)	Profit margin percentage	Estimated research and development expenditure ($ million)	Estimated expenditure on publicity and information ($ million)
1	Hoffmann-La Roche	Switzerland	3,100	19	400	300
2	Merck & Co	USA	2,200	28	170	230
3	Hoechst	Germany	2,000	18	160	280
4	Ciba-Geigy	Switzerland	1,800	21	150	220
5	Bayer	Germany	1,600	16	100	200
6	American Home Products	USA	1,500	24	50	150
7	Sandoz	Switzerland	1,400	17	180	200
8	Bristol-Myers	USA	1,400	18	90	210
9	Warner Lambert	USA	1,300	14	70	220
10	Pfizer	USA	1,300	23	100	170
11	Boehringer Ingelheim	Germany	1,300	28	120	210
12	Eli Lilly	USA	1,200	27	150	160
13	Upjohn	USA	1,100	19	120	130
14	Rhone-Poulenc	France	1,000	13	90	80
15	Takeda	Japan	1,000	18	80	90
16	Glaxo	UK	1,000	17	80	100
17	Smith Kline	USA	1,000	29	70	120
18	Squibb	USA	900	15	60	110
19	Schering-Plough	USA	900	28	70	130
20	Beecham	UK	800	22	50	100
21	Abbott	USA	800	20	60	90
22	Roussel Uclaf	France	700	11	50	80
23	Sterling Winthrop	USA	700	17	40	120
24	Schering (Berlin)	Germany	700	16	90	100
25	Johnson & Johnson	USA	700	24	80	120
26	Fujisawa	Japan	700	19	50	50
27	Montedison	Italy	600	5	30	40
28	Shionogi	Japan	600	13	60	70
29	ICI	UK	600	19	50	90
30	Akzo	Holland	600	11	60	80

Based on information presented at the Aries International Symposium, 'Competition in Multinational Drugs', held in Paris on 19th June, 1980, by Dr Robert Aries.

Pfizer has subsidiaries in Argentina, Australia, Belgium, Brazil, Canada, Chile, Colombia, England, France, Germany, Greece, India, Italy, Japan, Mexico, Nigeria, Pakistan, Philippines, Spain, Sri Lanka, Taiwan, Turkey, Venezuela and Zimbabwe.

Merck, Sharp & Dohme: Mr Merck's enterprise in its present form has subsidiaries in Argentina, Australia, Bermuda, Brazil, Canada, Colombia, England, France, Germany, Holland, Hong Kong, Italy, Japan, Mexico, Pakistan, Panama, Peru, Philippines, South Africa and Thailand.

Sterling has subsidiaries in Argentina, Australia, Brazil, Canada, Chile, Colombia, Costa Rica, Dominican Republic, Ecuador, El Salvador, England, France, Ghana, Guatemala, Honduras, Italy, Jamaica, Malaysia, Mexico, New Zealand, Nicaragua, Peru, Philippines, Puerto Rico, South Africa, Trinidad and Venezuela.

There can hardly be a country in the non-communist world that does not have at least one United States drug manufacturer's subsidiary. And where the Americans have gone, their Swiss, British and German rivals are sure to have followed. They go in search of even bigger profits, bigger markets, more economies of scale; and inevitably they gain immense political power along the way.

A characteristic feature of multinational companies is that their subsidiaries operate under the discipline of a common global strategy, within the framework of common global control. The head office is the brain and nerve centre. It evolves the corporate strategy, decides where new investment should be located, allocates export markets and research programmes to the subsidiaries, and determines prices and profits on all inter-affiliate exchanges. The options available to the multinational give it tremendous leverage when negotiating with governments, and it is very rare for the interests of the multinational to suffer in any conflict of interest. Countries are regarded as constituencies by the corporations, and the parts of the world that are open to them are crossed and divided with an intricate web of international agreements and licensing arrangements.[10] The different laws and regulations of each individual nation simply form a differently shaped container into which the same medicines are poured.

Despite the megalithic nature of the companies that control three-quarters of the drugs prescribed in the Western world, there is still some room for the small operator. The American company, Marion Laboratories Inc., began as a one-man business. It was started in the mid 1950s by Ewing Kauffman, described by *Fortune* magazine as a 'man who could sell rubber crutches'. Kauffman began by selling pills to doctors, a preparation called Vicam, which contained a mixture of vitamins and some chemicals said to 'detoxify the upper tract'. The company was started with $5,500, and Mr Kauffman has not looked back. Profits have rocketed, sales passed the $50 million mark in 1972 and shares in the company rose from $21 in 1965 to $636 in 1972. When Ewing Kauffman began, he was embarrassed about being a one-man business, so he gave the company his middle name to hide the fact. He bottled the pills in his basement, and when calling on doctors would swallow one, saying with pride that 'Vicam would detoxify his upper tract'. This seemed to work very well, but it did involve frequent interruptions to business as the pills had an unfortunate laxative effect.[11]

Another well-recognised characteristic of drug manufacturers and distributors, whatever their size, is their profitability. The attitude that underwrites the high profitability has been described by Dr Dale Console, a former medical director of E.R. Squibb & Co. He told a United States Senate sub-committee on monopoly in the drug industry: 'The pharmaceutical industry is unique in that it can make exploitation seem a noble purpose. It is the organised, carefully planned, and skilful execution of this exploitation that constitutes one of the costs of drugs which must be measured not only in terms of dollars, but in terms of the inroads the industry has made into the entire structure of medicine and medical care.'[12]

Whatever the other effects of the over-promotion of drugs, it is in dollars, pounds, francs and marks that the success of the commercial strategy of corporations is measured.

Shareholders like drug companies; they are good investments. Pre-tax profits are consistently higher than in other types of manufacturing industry, whatever swings or trends may affect the economy as a whole. A typical, though fictitious, drug manufacturer will have a profit and loss statement something like this:

Total sales revenue	100 per cent
from which deduct: Cost of manufacture	40
to give Gross profit margin:	60
From this deduct:	
Marketing costs,	15
Research and development, and	10
General and administrative costs	5
This gives a final Profit before tax of	30 per cent

In money terms, this sort of analysis can mean, as with Beecham in 1973, that pharmaceutical sales of £95 million brought almost £24 million trading profit.[13] Beecham's main contribution to the ethical drug field is one widely prescribed antibiotic, ampicillin, marketed under the brand name Penbritin.

From 1960 to 1972, United States drug manufacturers averaged 18 per cent net profit after tax, compared with 11 per cent for all United States manufacturing corporations. The average profit on sales was over 9 per cent, compared with less than 6 per cent for other industry. These figures actually *underestimate* the profitability of drug manufacturing because many drug companies also market other products on which profits are less; and many companies have established operations in countries such as Puerto Rico where they can achieve net profits as high as 40 per cent after tax.[14]

The industry claims that high profits are necessary because this business is typified by high risk and strong competition, with high quality control and research costs. The last two items are passed on in the price of drugs, so is there adequate justification for such profits in terms of risk? Not according to the United States Government's Task Force on Prescription Drugs, who stated quite emphatically that 'the exceptionally high rate of profit which generally marks the drug industry is not accompanied by any particular degree of risk or by any unique difficulties in obtaining growth capital'.[15]

Nor is there justification for the claim that the industry is competitive. It is not, as the Kefauver hearings concluded. In 1959, Estes Kefauver and his staff in the Senate Subcommittee on Antitrust and Monopoly began an investigation into the pharmaceutical industry. Searching for information, Senator Kefauver issued subpoenas to the top drug manufacturers in the United States. The response was immediate: the senator was assailed as a 'coonskinhatted hillbilly publicity seeker and an enemy of free enterprise'.[16] Undeterred by pressure to quash the investigation, Kefauver conducted hearings which revealed a host of unsavoury practices in the industry. One finding was that the structure of the market allows the appearance of competition when it is absent. No company has more than 10 per cent of the market, and the industry argues that this is obvious evidence of competition. However, it is a divided market. Each company has its speciality, and ICI's heart pills do not complete with Beecham's antibiotics or Roche's tranquillizers. Kefauver found that of fifty-one chemical entities comprising two-thirds of United States prescription sales, twenty-seven had only one producer, eight had two, ten had three, and none had more than seven. This situation underlines the high concentration of production and marketing around non-competing specialities.[17]

In most industries, lower prices for similar products give a competitive edge which can be decisive for sales and therefore for profits. The pharmaceutical market, however, is remarkably insensitive to price, whereas the profit made by a drug is very sensitive to it. This is illustrated clearly for the typical company shown below, if all the factors are altered by 10 per cent. It will be seen that a 10 per cent price increase brings far greater rewards to the company than any other sort of increase or economy.

The lesson is obvious. It is always worthwhile to keep prices high and back each product with heavy promotions, which will in all probability be paid for by an increase in sales volume, despite the 'high' price.[18] This is confirmed by the US Health, Education, and Welfare task force finding that the pharmaceutical industry is prepared to spend anywhere from 15 to 35 per cent of its sales income on marketing, roughly three times the level of United States manufacturing in general.[19]

Factor altered	percentage increase in profit before tax
10 per cent increase in price	33
10 per cent increase in sales volume	20
10 per cent decrease in manufacturing costs	13
10 per cent decrease in marketing expenditure	5
10 per cent decrease in research expenditure	3
10 per cent decrease in general and admin. expenditure	2

As price has more effect on profit than anything else, it is not surprising that companies will at times go to extraordinary lengths to avoid reducing it. In the late 1960s, Hoffmann-La Roche were under pressure from the British government, who felt that they were making excessive profits from the National Health Service. Rather than reduce the price of their drugs, the company gave back to the government £1.6 million in compensation for excess profits. This was more acceptable to Roche than straight price cuts, as cuts in Britain would immediately bring the company under pressure to cut prices in all their other markets. It has been argued that the selfish attitude of the British government helped to keep prices up around the world.[20]

As a further alternative to price cuts, Roche gave Valium gratis to British hospitals, a tactic they were to repeat in Canada.[21] This nice gesture created a market for Valium among patients during after-care, and through the trainee doctors' habitual prescribing of the drug.

In 1970, when Roche refunded £900,000 to the National Health Service, the Monopolies Commission estimated that Roche had made £4 million profit on sales of £6.8 million of Librium and Valium in Britain; although at the time, by adjusting the buying and selling prices between head office and subsidiary of various material and agreement contents, Roche arrived at a profit figure of only £500,000.[22]

The prices of name brand drugs are whatever the market will stand,[23] [24] and therefore can have little to do with rational cost factors. Through heavy promotion, companies aim to achieve 'a monopoly of reputation' or medical habit, which ensures that expensive branded drugs are prescribed almost exclusively, even when generic equivalents are available. One example will suffice to illustrate the result of this strategy. When Schering were selling Meticorten for $102.57 per 1,000 tablets, a generic version of the same drug, prednisone USP, was available for $4.40 per 1,000.[25]

This situation is a consequence of the system of patent protection for new drugs. Patents prevent competitors from copying new products and selling them to the detriment of the inventor, who may have invested a lot of time and money. When a new drug appears, it can be produced only by the patent-holder, or by licensing arrangement agreed with him. The patent-holder's brand will dominate the market and fix the price.

The successful operation of multinational drug companies depends on the international acknowledgement of their patent rights. Although there is no international patent system as such, the International Convention for the Protection of Industrial Property lays down basic principles to which member countries must conform. These include equal and reciprocal treatment and recognition in patent matters for nationals of each member country, provision for determining the date when the patent was filed, and conditions for licensing foreign-owned patents. Within a broad framework, the International Convention was content to leave the signatories to the agreement ample scope within which to adapt the details of patents in keeping with national requirements.[26] Any attempt to alter patent law in any way which could be detrimental to their interests is naturally resisted vigorously by the drug companies.

In addition to protecting the market for a product, the patent system allows multinationals to develop where technology is cheap, manufacture where materials and labour are cheap, and sell where the market is rich.

The possession of patent rights in a drug has a further valuable result. The patent holder has a unique control over the information given to the users of the drug, doctors and pharmacists, and this increases his power over the market.

In the United States, the authoritative reference book on drugs is the *Physician's Desk Reference (PDR)*, which is published each year by Medical Economics Inc. It is supplied free to doctors, and contains information about prescription drugs produced by members of the Pharmaceutical Manufacturer's Association. The entry on each drug is quite comprehensive and must be agreed with the government Bureau of Drugs. But it is in the way the information is ordered that the PDR is made particularly useful to the industry. It is arranged alphabetically by the name of the manufacturing company, and then by the brand name of the product. This forces the doctor to learn brand name and manufacturer for any drug about which he seeks further information – and so brand loyalty is encouraged. If the doctor tries to start by diagnosing a condition and then seeking an appropriate treatment, he is lost. The gaps in the system are bridged by advertising material and detailmen who keep the company and the product name foremost in his mind.

In Britain, too, doctors rely on drug reference material which is controlled by the pharmaceutical industry. The most widely used source is MIMS (Monthly Index of Medical Specialities),[27] which, like the PDR, is a compendium of material supplied by drug manufacturers. MIMS is designed for convenience: pocket-sized and organised in a highly access-ible way, with a therapeutic index, trade-name equivalents of generic drugs and a brand-name index. The main text is categorised according to the use of the drugs, grouped under system headings such as 'cardio-vascular system', and sub-sections with headings such as 'antibiotics', 'oral contraceptives', 'antihypertensives' and 'sedatives and tranquillizers'.

MIMS gives little precise information on when particular drugs should be used, or when they should be avoided. Contrary to the beliefs of many British doctors, it rarely warns of adverse reactions. These are described in a second publication produced by the industry, the second most used source of information: the Data Sheet Compendium. It is organised in much the same way as the PDR, but without the same wealth of detail. But even here some adverse drug reactions are not mentioned, especially those caused by older drugs for which data sheets do not have to be approved by government; and mentions are often made in such a way that the effect of the warning may be lost and prescribers may be lulled into a false sense of security about drug safety. An example will illustrate the technique; the following warnings are the most extensive given for progestogens which are proposed for use during pregnancy, and which have repeatedly been implicated in the production of congenital mal-formations.

Proluton Depot
Warnings: Many medicinal products, including female sex hormones, have been suspected of being capable of affecting the normal develop-ment of a child in the early stages of pregnancy. Many researchers consider that in relation to sex hormones such a suspicion is ill founded but one has to accept that for no medicinal product can a teratogenic activity be excluded with absolute certainty. Therefore, the general principle is now widely accepted that the inessential use of drugs during pregnancy should be avoided.[28]

Drug companies pay a fee for inclusion in the Data Sheet Compendium, and some smaller manufacturers are left out. MIMS, in contrast, is comprehensive, with listings financed by the sale of advertising space. Different versions are published for different parts of the world, and the drug companies have no problems in giving different information about the same drug for different markets, at times to a bizarre and dangerous degree.

MIMS Africa includes drugs which are not to be found in MIMS UK because they are deemed too hazardous. One such group is the dipyrones, analgesics related to aspirin which can cause fatal blood disease. Winthrop's Conmel (500 mg dipyrone) is given simply as 'Analgesic, antipyretic, anti-rheumatic'; while Hoechst's Cantacin, a curious mixture which includes a type of dipyrone, is offered for 'Feverish colds, influenzal infections'. No warnings appear for either preparation, although neither can be sold in Britain, the United States or most other developed countries. Where there are fewer controls, unacceptably dangerous drugs bring further profits for the drug companies.

Given virtually unrestricted opportunities, the multinational pharmaceutical companies put tremendous marketing effort into third world countries. Some of those with British factories have earned the prestigious

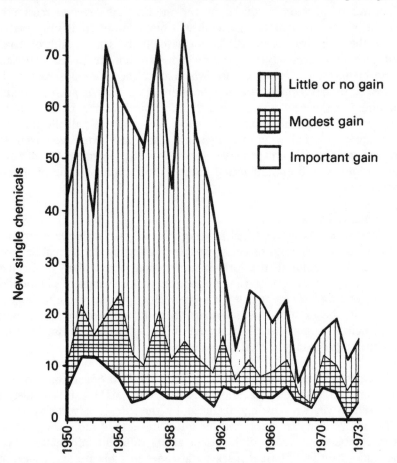

Diagram 1. Annual approvals of new drugs by degree of therapeutic gain. United States 1950–73.

Source: A.M. Schmidt, statement to Senate Sub-Committee on Health (1974). Reproduced from Steward, F., Ref. 31.

Queen's Award to Industry for their export achievements. The Director General of the World Health Organisation has preferred to label them with some bitterness as 'drug colonialists'.[29]

Predictably, the regulations in the affluent countries are resented by the pharmaceutical industry. George Teeling-Smith, director of the industry-sponsored Office of Health Economics in Britain, expressed attitudes characteristic of the industry when he commented: 'We are a highly regulated industry, but as far as drug safety is concerned the amount of regulation is certainly not inadequate, in our view I think it is excessive, and in particular it produces too much in the way of requirements before

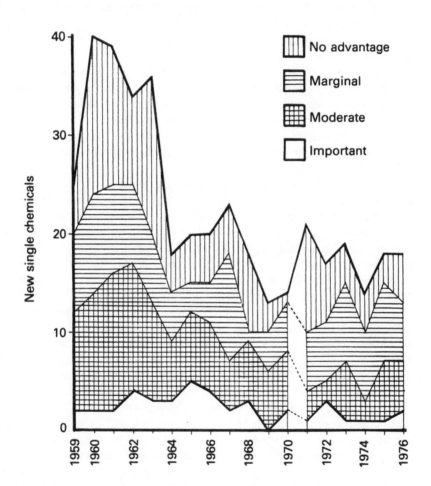

Diagram 2. New drugs marketed per year according to therapeutic significance, Britain 1959–76. Reproduced from Steward, F., Ref. 31.

the first trial of the drug in man. And I think in turn this tends to inhibit research by discouraging research in areas where there is need for a new drug, but where the cost of development would be prohibitive.'[30]

These claims do not stand up to scrutiny. Studies in Britain[31] and the United States[32] have shown that regulations, far from 'discouraging research in areas where there is need for a new drug', have served only to prevent the repetitive marketing of similar drugs and to reduce the number of combination products. The decline of new chemical entities has been slight, and indeed is to be expected in view of the intensity of research effort over the past three decades.

In the United States, there has been very little change in the rate of introduction of new drugs which represent an important therapeutic gain since 1955, although the numbers offering little or no advantage have dropped sharply.[33]

Perhaps the confusion revolves around the question of *whose* needs new products serve. Behind statements like Teeling-Smith's lies the implication that we, consumers and governments, must be sympathetic to drug manufacturers or we won't get the medicines we need. Reassuringly, as we shall see, the evidence points to the conclusion that we can well afford controls because the effect is to save us from many medicines that we certainly don't need.

The drug regulation issue is one part of the question of the relationship between the industry and government. It is a relationship where the government is all too often on the losing side. To the multinational drug manufacturer, governments fall into two broad categories, those dependent on subsidiaries and imports for their medicinal needs, and those with their own indigenous industry which exports drugs. The former include most poor Third World countries, where the government's total budget may be only a fraction of that of the multinational corporation with which it is dealing. The local subsidiary may try to harmonise its objectives with those of the locality, and may be prepared to undertake the occasional loss-leader venture for the sake of goodwill.[34] But this will not alter the fact that it has an over-riding extra-national commitment to its parent company, and that the parent has the power to enforce that commitment.

Governments with their own indigenous industry are little better placed. They are caught in a classic political/economic trap. The electorate in a democratic country demands limits to the freedom permitted to drug manufacturers, so regulations are necessary and governments must devise and enforce them. But the same government desperately wants the balance of payments earnings and tax generated by the pharmaceutical trade.

While taxes are not a matter for negotiation, regulations are; and battles are fought against them on a more or less continuous basis. The West German state, for example, earned about DM3,700 million ($2,083 million) from taxes paid by the drug supply system in 1978. This was broken down as follows: DM965 million in taxes from the industry (on a production value of DM13,400 million); DM1,000 million from wholesalers and pharmacists; DM1,600 million in value added tax; and DM,100 million tax on alcohol used by the industry.[35] Is it coincidental that the West German pharmaceutical industry is more free of regulation than the US equivalent, where the state takes a much smaller proportion of its earnings in tax?

In most countries, the drug manufacturers have formed trade associations which act as powerful lobbies for the industry's interests. In the United States there is the Pharmaceutical Manufacturers' Association, in Germany the Bundesverband der Pharmazeutischen Industrie. Britain has the Association of British Pharmaceutical Industries. And so on. The Pharmaceutical Manufacturers' Association in the United States has a record of successful resistance to what it regards as unfavourable legislative changes, and it is supported in many of its battles with government by the prestigious and powerful American Medical Association. The close alliance of these two bodies is underlined by the fact that a recent president of the PMA, Joseph Stetler, was formerly general counsel to the AMA for twelve years. The AMA is an associate member of the Pharmaceutical Manufacturers' Association.[36]

State medicine, in the form of the National Health Service in Britain, serves to focus both the government's dichotomy of interest and its inability to cope with the pharmaceutical industry even when it is in an overwhelmingly good commercial bargaining position. In a situation parallel to that in America, the pharmaceutical industry in Britain counts on the British Medical Association to support its interests; but its main power-base is the Association of British Pharmaceutical Industries, the ABPI. To illustrate the political power and penetration by the pharmaceutical industry under conditions that should favour their adversaries, we shall look at the development of the ABPI and its relationship with successive British governments.

The roots of the ABPI go back to 1867, although its modern history starts in 1930 with the formation of the Wholesale Drug Trade Association (WDTA), from which the ABPI was to emerge in June 1948, one month before the launch of the National Health Service. British drug trade associations have a long tradition of close involvement in political questions. At its foundation the precursor of the ABPI adopted the specific objective, 'to represent the views of the trade in all matters affecting its interests and to promote or oppose . . . departmental or parliamentary legislation affecting the trade'.[37]

The first apparent threat from government to the pharmaceutical industry came in 1946, when the post-war socialist, or Labour, administration nationalised the railways and mines. This brought fear of a similar fate to every major industry, and in its annual report of 1946 the WDTA prepared to meet this threat:

> The Council has been conscious of the high responsibility that rests upon the British pharmaceutical industry as an indispensible component of the National Health Service. Firmly believing that the industry itself, by its own insight, experience, and endeavours, can best maintain and promote its own efficiency, the Council has been engaged upon a draft revision of the Constitution and rules of the Association with a view to enlarging the scope while maintaining the quality of membership and giving formal recognitions to the social obligations of the industry.[38]

In 1950, the Ministry of Health first showed anxiety about the growing bill for prescription drugs. A circular was sent to doctors asking them not to prescribe brand name drugs unless no alternative was available. This circular, like the many that were to follow, had little effect; it was merely the opening shot in a campaign against drug costs which was to be waged by successive Labour and Conservative governments in the years to come.

During the 1950s, government investigations into drug costs forced the ABPI to set up a high-geared public relations exercise 'which would bring home to the general public the . . . achievements of pharmaceutical private enterprise'. It seems to have succeeded. In 1959, the president of the ABPI was able to comment: 'The industry had not so far had to face the threat of hostile legislation [and] . . . it was well aware that a quietly conducted . . . campaign based on the simple premise that the industry was doing a good job might well forestall or mitigate legislation.'[39]

But in fact it was a Conservative Minister of Health, Enoch Powell, who shattered the complacency of the ABPI by importing cheap drugs from abroad. The ABPI was forced to learn quickly that a free-enterprise political philosophy could make an excellent case for lower drug costs. And whereas previously the pharmaceutical industry had nestled comfortably under Conservative governments, it was now uneasy and sceptical of any administration.

Powell's action led to an immediate intensification of the ABPI public relations campaign. At this time, the opposition Labour party was led by Harold Wilson, who proposed in 1961 that 'the Health Service meets its needs increasingly from public enterprise, either by provision through new publicly owned undertakings or by the acquisition of existing ones; that the patents covering some of these drugs be thrown open for the use of the State'.[40] Strong medicine, in no way sweetened when Wilson became Prime Minister in 1964.

But for all the socialist sabre-rattling in opposition, the only tangible evidence of conviction in office was another enquiry, by the Sainsbury Committee. And by this time, the ABPI had matured. Its Nationalisation Study Group had spawned four sub-groups, able to answer questions posed by parliamentary critics. By 1965, the ABPI was a sophisticated and powerful political organisation, capable of meeting the many complex stresses which a National Health Service placed on it.

In 1970 the ABPI was considered by Laurie Pavitt MP, then chairman of the Parliamentary Labour Party's Committee on Health, to be the third most powerful – although the most discreet – pressure group in Britain. He ranked it after the Trades Union Council and the National Farmers' Union, but before the Confederation of British Industry.

How was the ABPI able to thrive through twenty years of legislative threats and growing government disquiet about drug costs? The answer can be traced to a classic British compromise, the introduction of a Voluntary Price Regulation Scheme. After three years of negotiation, in 1957, a scheme proposed by the ABPI for regulating the prices of branded prescription drugs on the basis of 'acceptable profits' was accepted by the government. The ABPI issued a public statement: 'This will end a lot of the criticisms that prices are excessive.'

The Voluntary Price Regulation Scheme (VPRS) worked on a constant negotiation, compromise and agreement basis between the ABPI and the government. It brought the two bodies ever closer together, in a profitable dance of mutual understanding in which neither partner could leave the floor. The intimacy of this working relationship enabled the ABPI to resist the many pressures that have been put on it over the years.

Although the scheme was theoretically a voluntary one, it came to be treated as obligatory by both sides, and as time passed, the fortunes and interests of one side were becoming progressively more dependent upon, and identical with, those of the other.

There is no doubt, however, that the ABPI remained extremely sensitive to public criticism. Each move by government against pharmaceutical industry interests was countered not only by the lobbying of numerous well-briefed committees behind the scenes, but also by a marked increase in expenditure on public relations.

Seeking to 'create a personality with the general public', the ABPI sought every opportunity to make a showing on radio, TV and in national newspapers. At one point it even considered the possibility of a TV soap opera with a drug industry background. The high point of the campaign in the 1960s was when the ABPI president spoke on BBC Radio's *Woman's Hour* about the safety of drugs with Sir Derrick Dunlop, then Chairman of the Committee on Safety of Drugs. The success of the ABPI's various strategies may be judged from the fact that, so soon after the thalidomide tragedy, the industry looked upon Sir Derrick as an industry representative.[41]

If the ABPI acts, as it were, as the army defending the pharmaceutical industry, then it has its own undercover intelligence operation. This is the official-sounding Office of Health Economics, founded by the ABPI in 1962.

The major function of the Office of Health Economics (OHE) is to create a favourable public image. To do this, it liaises with the press, produces attractive and well-written publications, assists selected research projects and involves itself in 'education', especially of general practitioners.

OHE publications project two recurring messages. First, that research by drug manufacturers must be maintained and not jeopardised by governments; and second, that drugs are not expensive, either in absolute terms or in relation to the price of care in other sectors of the health service. Penetration is achieved because the OHE does publish some very good material on health. Laurie Pavitt argued that 90 per cent of its publications are excellent while 10 per cent are outright propaganda. This is public relations at its most skilful because people are willing to accept the 10 per cent for the sake of the 90 per cent. If the ratio were changed the plausibility would be diminished. According to Sir Derrick Dunlop, the publications are 'little masterpieces'.[42]

The OHE has its own press and political network. Politicians, the press and TV researchers rely on the OHE for information and comment on current health topics, and the more this happens, the greater is the success of the whole extravagant public relations exercise. And this is what it is about: convincing individuals and institutions throughout society as a whole that drugs are good, the drug industry is good and what is good for them is bound to be good for you.

This examination of the relationships between the pharmaceutical industry and its political, social and economic environment, and of its efforts to control and manipulate that environment, has focused on Britain. But the same mechanisms are active to a greater or lesser degree in every country.

When multinational drug companies join together in association their power can be overwhelming. They can change or resist the intention of the legislative process by applying their power to government, and they can maintain the commercial interests of their industry over any rational medical need for their products. They have deliberately created myths about the power, potential, and beneficial effects of their medicines that are extremely dangerous. In the third world countries, sales pressure from the drug manufacturers sucks up resources and trained personnel that could be more constructively and cost-effectively used in basic primary health care.

The possession of power and influence on this scale is not tempered by real public accountability or by an inherent code of ethics. Multinational corporations exist to make profits. Medical practitioners are concerned with healing. Are they compatible bedfellows? A classic graffiti-artist's slogan suggests the answer: 'The makers of aspirin wish you had a headache right now.'

Chapter Five

Good Business Sense

What makes good business sense to a multinational drug company?

Ideally it would be to find a cheaply made drug, which has the following virtues:

1 It must be protected by world-wide patents.
2 It must be suitable for world-wide promotion.
3 It should create a mild psychological dependence in its users.
4 It should give the appearance of answering some expressed medical need.
5 It should not produce unmanageable side-effects.

The last requirement is more significant that it might at first appear. With manageable side-effects emerging from a drug with an established market, the lucky manufacturer can go back to his laboratory to find a suitable cure for these unfortunate, unforeseen, but unavoidable, occurrences.

In the previous chapter we illustrated the fact that price is the key factor in the profitability of a drug business. It was also clear that it was far better strategy to spend money on promoting a drug to maintain sales, than to reduce the price to increase the market. The result has been the development of an industry that is known for its sustained aggressive marketing and promotion throughout the world. On the international scale this has inevitably led to the reduction of people and disease conditions to so many millions of classifiable potential sales units. One persistent, old-fashioned idea must be examined against the essentially commercial nature of drug manufacturing. It is that drugs are developed in response to knowledge of a disease in order to provide a cure. Many years ago, when the major scourges were still everyday causes of death, and knowledge of chemistry was embryonic, this was probably true. But today the illness–treatment sequence has effectively been reversed. Increasingly, the treatment is discovered, and a suitable illness identified, or promoted, to comply with it.

Over the past decade the pharmaceutical industry has moved into new growth areas where the success of their products depends implicitly on a cultural acceptance of their public relations message. As we shall see in the following chapter, the benefits of the use of their products are assumed, very rarely proved. Before illustrating some of the ways in which drug manufacturers are proceeding with what has been described as the medicalisation of society, we shall briefly examine the way the industry uses conventional marketing techniques to underwrite the sale of their products.

Advertising sells drugs in the same way that it sells anything else. The medical profession is reached by series advertisements which support the numerous publications that make up the specialised medical press. A high proportion of pages will be devoted to advertising copy that is lavish, colourful, slickly produced and very persistent. Most medical publications exist purely on this wealth of advertising revenue; for example it brings the *Journal of the American Medical Association* seven million dollars each year.[1] This must inevitably affect editorial outlook.[2] There are various special codes of practice, or regulations, which control drug advertising copy, usually bearing on the factual content. Typically this will consist of details of the presentation of the drug, that is, its forms and packaging, the clinical indications for which it should be prescribed, dosage recommendations, any contra-indications or conditions which would make its use inadvisable, specific cautions and any frequent acknowledged adverse reactions.[3]

The factual information tends to be printed in very small type, whereas the commercial or fantasy message may be in letters inches high. The old advertising rule, 'he who runs must be able to read' is particularly apt for busy physicians, and the design is such that they can hardly miss the key words. For example, Smith, Kline & French used a full-page advertisement in various medical magazines with four outstanding words in bright red: OLDER PATIENTS – ANTIHYPERTENSIVES – DYAZIDE. The accompanying three column inches of small black type will only reach those with better eyesight, more time or a special interest.

Even in this area there may be pitfalls for the unwary. Within the medical press a form of cosy commercial incest underlies the small print of drug advertisements. Frequently claims made for a drug are legitimised by reference to research papers published in medical journals. Most doctors who glance at those references undoubtedly assume that the papers have appeared in journals like the *British Medical Journal*, whose editors submit every paper offered to detailed scrutiny by expert referees to weed out poorly designed or worthless research. But drug companies do not publish many of their findings in such respected journals. Often they are published without such scrutiny in journals which charge fees for printing work of this nature.

The Journal of International Medical Research, for example, was charging £85 per page for publishing scientific papers in 1975. When Vernon Coleman, a medical writer and general practitioner, wrote to ICI for information on their antidepressant Vivalan, he was sent a 'typically colourful and well-produced brochure describing in the usual glowing terms the work done, proving how effective and unique Vivalan is'. The majority of the references quoted in support of this 'vivid prose' had been published in the *Journal of International Medical Research*.[4]

Prescription drugs are not advertised openly to the public. But obviously it would be advantageous if the public were made aware of what was available, what they could expect, or demand, from their physicians. Hence from the PR machine stream breathlessly excited news items recognisable by the key clichés which the media find acceptable: 'new drug' heralds another 'amazing breakthrough' which, 'after years of research', is a 'weapon in the battle against' a disease; the 'miracle drug brings new hope to sufferers'; and so on. Cooperation in these exercises may be encouraged by various means. Sandoz flew a bevy of journalists to Switzerland, where hospitality broke out, on the occasion of the launch of their therapeutically unremarkable anti-asthma drug Zaditen.[5] Everyone who read a newspaper in Britain must have been aware of the virtues and availability of the new drug.

Doctors also receive sales literature directly from drug companies. It is often a matter of complaint; the sheer quantity of paper makes it totally overwhelming. Some of it is no doubt very informative, perhaps even helpful, but every piece is designed to sell a particular product. The content varies from the single-sheet blunt prod: 'Migraine? Prescribe . . .', through pseudo-personal letters, the 'Dear Doctors', and messages on golf balls, diaries, table mats and other minor items, to lavish reference works and impressive 'educational' or 'post-graduate' courses.[6] The resources used to produce this mountain of promotional material, and the cost of circulating it, are phenomenal.

Finally, but most important, the physician is confronted by the drug company's detailmen, its super sales representatives. Their job is to promote the use of and to sell ethical drugs and other pharmaceutical products to physicians, dentists, hospitals and retail and wholesale drug establishments. To do this they need to have and to utilise knowledge of medical practices, drugs and medicines, and be able to inform their customers of new drugs, explain therapeutic characteristics and clinical studies conducted with drugs and to discuss dosage, use and effect of new drugs and other medical preparations.

Dr Dale Console has written: 'The primary purpose of the detailman is to make a sale, even if it involves irrational prescribing and irrational combinations.' And he has summarised the technique involved as: 'If you can't convince them, confuse them.'[7]

The detailman's primary target is the prescribing physician, to whose desk he directs a flow of product and development information, samples, news of recent clinical discoveries, and reinforcing gossip of what other similar physicians are doing – that is, happily prescribing his company's products. More insidiously, he may spread tales of failure or doubt of other companies' drugs. These tales have been proved untrue so often that in America the FDA has been forced to take steps to counter the practice. Detailmen have spread rumours of therapeutic failure with generic equivalents of their branded products when no such failures have occurred. Conversely they have offered reassurance on the safety of particular drugs, when such selective reassurance has been totally unjustified.[8]

The classic example of 'selective detailing' is provided by Eli Lilly. Their antibiotic erythromycin estolate, sold as Ilosone, was producing a much greater rate of adverse reactions than other erythromycins. It was showing around a twenty-fold increase in liver damage and producing jaundice in between one and 14 per cent of users. Its benefits were therefore dubious.

Nevertheless Lilly continued to promote Ilosone through their detailmen. According to an internal company document:

> Ilosone is favoured by regular users mainly because of their loyalty to Lilly . . . Ilosone is not substantially differentiated from other erythromycins (by physicians). Thus, Lilly can promote Ilosone as an erythromycin which conveys safety . . . A delicate balance is required so as not to raise unnecessary concern among those physicians who are not generally concerned about the jaundice problem.
>
> Selective detailing may be required to avoid discussion of Ilosone with any physician who is aware and concerned about liver toxicity side effects. Where there is any awareness of Ilosone's liver toxicity associations, the known availability of a 'safe alternative like Erythrocin' is competitively decisive.

The market study from which these quotations are taken went on to say that not many physicians were aware of Ilosone's liver toxicity 'associations'. Consequently during 1971 the safer Erythrocin, produced by

Abbott's, sold $28 million, while Ilosone sold $27 million. By 1978 Ilosone had 25 per cent of the erythromycin market, over $61 million, despite a prominent warning on the package label and a drug bulletin alert issued in 1974 by the FDA.[9]

Detailmen also call on wholesale pharmacists, to make sure supply levels are adequate and to maintain goodwill. Their routine is repeated with the dispensing pharmacist, although in a lower key. The most important task is the location of physicians who may not be prescribing the company's lines adequately. The detailmen can then call on the physician to overcome resistance, perhaps by an invitation to a conference or seminar, with golf, food and excellent wine thrown in as required. Through the pharmacist the detailman may also be able to identify the high prescribers; these are particularly valuable because they show maximum brand loyalty.[10] In this way the loops are closed and market pressure maintained.

In 1975 in the United States there were 26,500 detailmen calling on 200,000 physicians and 7,000 hospitals. They accounted for 55 per cent of the total sales expenditure of the pharmaceutical industry, around $36,000 each per annum, or a total of $955 million overall.[11]

In countries where the market is more open, less subject to the distinct boundaries provided by professional and regulatory standards, the company rep can come into his own. For example in Tanzania there is one detailman for every four doctors. This situation is regretted by the authorities, because of the loss of human resources. It is the good paramedics who become the reps, and instead of participating in basic healing processes they help the flood of unnecessary, unsuitable and expensive drugs that distort the pattern of care. The flood is complemented by the vacuum cleaner effect that the successful promotion of drugs has, in taking money directly from the economy, where it could be better used in the improvement of health by providing basics like more clean water and sewage treatment. In India, where Boots and Glaxo have between them more representatives than the government has drug inspectors, the sheer weight of numbers can keep a market wide open.[12]

Patients rarely see anything of this enormous sales effort, although they may meet the detailman without realising who he is. A letter to the *New England Journal of Medicine* from a young doctor describes an 'advanced training program for "the informed pharmaceutical representative".' She tells how detailmen are assigned to hospital interns on their morning ward rounds. They can make their sales pitch from a 'distinctive vantage point – the patient's bedside'. She continues, 'are we not, by allowing such activities (often for fees), making commercial salesmen privy to the private lives of our patients so that they can better market their drugs? Are these patients made aware that one of the white coated figures at the bedside is not a physician or a medical student and is not bound by a physician's oath to serve that patient's best interest?"[13]

Britain has fewer drug representatives, 1,200 to 25,000 general practitioners.[14] In the United States only about one-fifth of the physicians in private practice are GPs, but this 40,000 provides the cream; the top prescribers are there.

The top one per cent may prescribe as much as ten times the average. The more uniform rate of prescribing in Britain, where the average physician writes 1,000 prescriptions per month, and the top one per cent only manage around 3,000, is ascribed by the industry to the lack of financial incentive for the British doctor to see more patients.[15]

To focus the firepower of advertising, literature and detailmen on their target, the physician, the drug companies spend enormous amounts of money. In 1975 in the United States the industry spent 22 per cent of its sales revenue on this armoury, or $1,820 million.[16] The table[17] below shows that this is not excessive in terms of developed countries.

Country	Promotion percentage of Sales
United States	22
West Germany	22
Italy	22
South Africa	22
Belgium	21
Canada	21
Sweden	18
India	18
France	17
Turkey	16
Indonesia	16
Britain	15

Concerned with problems of over-prescribing, various authorities have questioned this expenditure. One of the principle justifications of the drug industry is that it is necessary in order to educate the doctors and inform them of the vast range of pharmaceutical developments that are happening all the time. Dr Dale Console gave a more accurate perspective to a US Monopoly Subcommittee when he said:

How can legitimate education compete with the carefully contrived distortions driven home by the trip-hammer effect of weekly mailings, the regular visits of the detail man, two page spreads, and the ads that appear six times in the same journal; not to mention the added inducement of the free cocktail party and the golf outing complete with three golf balls stamped with the name of the doctor and company in contrasting colours? Drug advertising and promotion efforts encourage the doctor to believe that there is an easy way to practise medicine.[18]

Thus 'education' is the key rationalisation for the activities of detailmen and for much of the promotional effort directed at doctors. But the distortion of education passes beyond the surgery right into the academic institutions that shape medical attitudes. This penetration is achieved through sponsorship.

Sponsorship is regarded as a sound long-term investment by drug companies. It is arguably the most perverse form of generosity. It would be a labour beyond the strength of Hercules to discover with accuracy exactly how much research, in hospitals and universities, by professors, departmental heads, consultants, specialists, physicians, pharmacologists and other academics, is carried out with drug company money. Similarly, it is impossible to know how many people in prominent positions, medical professionals, academics, politicians and journalists, are engaged by the industry as advisers and consultants.[19] The whole stable is simply too big.

Active collaboration with the pharmaceutical industry is the rule in university pharmacology departments. This policy is hotly defended as mutually beneficial by the parties concerned,[20] yet inevitably it must threaten objectivity, the core concept of academic research. When a department head might lose half his staff if drug company support were withdrawn, he is likely to be more concerned about his status and career than worried about biased research.

While the front line sales battle rages around the world at the level of the doctors' consulting rooms, longer-term strategy is ordered from the more elevated vantage point of drug company executives. At this level, the key concept is 'competition', but as we have seen, drug manufacturers avoid competing directly with each other to supply a defined market for their product. Rather like athletes competing against the clock, their competition is to extend the market, to make the cake bigger. To this end, a variety of strategies which can be illustrated in terms of games have emerged which include some very opportunist but logical moves.

The first game is leapfrog. In conventional commercial leapfrog, salesmen working for the same company hop over each other and change territories. Each explains to the other's customers that things will be much better now that old so-and-so has gone, and using each other's customer reports they proceed to fill the gaps and wring the most out of the market.

Simple drug leapfrog is similar, except that the players stay still and the products leap over each other. After a time an established medication may begin to flag a little in the market, so a new form of exactly the same product is brought out, only this time it is yellow, instead of pink. The 'new' product is then run against the market of the old, with the aid of advertisements claiming that it is new and improved, even better than before. Add some conceptual trivia, such as 'A more convenient shape', or 'easier to take' and the game is on. Yellow will leap over pink in the market percentages, and should pick up new sales on the way.

There is a more complex game of drug leapfrog which is more serious and competitive. It involves an adversary and is a specialised game for the manufacturers of antibiotics. In an earlier chapter we described the problems that medicine encountered in trying to combat the effects of infections once the causative organism had entered the body. Penicillin changed that, but even at the height of its success, resistant strains of bacteria were beginning to appear. This provides the background to this form of leapfrog, which has gone roughly like this. With penicillin, nearly all the pathogens were killed, but some survived and adapted. The broad-spectrum antibiotics leapfrogged pencillin, and the process was repeated; then a new generation of narrow-spectrum specific antibiotics, such as lincomycin, leapfrogged the broad-spectrum drugs, and once more the process was repeated. Next came the broad-spectrum cephalosporins. Now it has been announced that an augmented form of pencillin has become available that prevents resistant bacteria from producing penicillinase. And so the game goes on, pathogens survive and adapt and new antibiotics are created.

Healthy resistant and adaptive pathogens mean a continuing healthy antibiotic market. To this end some bacteria oblige with little fuss. The gonococcus, the organism which causes gonorrhoea, plays the adversary very well. The popular Second World War variety had become 'Tokyo Rose', equally popular but penicillin-resistant, by the end of the Korean War, and the conflict in Vietnam produced the latest strain, against which very few antibiotics are effective. In this it was aided and abetted by the United States government. According to *New Republic*, 6th March 1971, 'in order to shore up Parke-Davis' declining chloramphenicol profits, the United States Defence Department purchased 10 million capsules for the South Vietnamese army and civilians, to be used in the usual indiscriminate manner'. Obliquely the free and easy use of the same antibiotics in factory farming is producing the same danger, this time from a super salmonella to poison us via the food chain.[21]

The innovative and enterprising nature of the pharmaceutical industry will no doubt maintain confidence in its ability to produce the goods at the appropriate time to keep these bacterial developments firmly in their place. That is, just one jump ahead of antibiotics, as profitable adversaries.

'Name games' are also important. As we have seen, naming drugs is a complex business. This complexity is exploited to the full by the industry. Thousands of drugs are available in different countries, each of which may have many brand names, many forms and many strengths. Periodically review bodies, committees or commissions naively suggest that this complexity should be reduced, and that doctors should prescribe by generic names.[22] Any such suggestion is emphatically rejected by the industry because complexity works to their advantage.

Attraction by association offers an apparent escape from the confusions of names. Doctors readily remember brand names which are similar to trusted names, so where a familiar niche has been created for a product it is sensible to make maximum use of it. Thiazide diuretics were the first effective and fairly safe ones available, and they have become synonymous with antihypertensive therapy. Smith, Kline & French chose the name Dyazide for their new diuretic. It is so close to thiazide that it will be readily remembered and quickly trusted. But the discrepancy is just enough to allow valid points of difference to be made to the doctor. The success of this strategy is reflected in Dyazide's rapid climb to the position of United States brand leader in 1980 in dollar value. Burroughs Wellcome's brand of digoxin, Lanoxin, and Squibb's fungicide Nystan (nystatin) are some of the hundreds of available examples.

A variation of the game is that of reflected use. Pfizer called its antidiabetic, chlorpropamide, Diabinese. And Glaxo's branded combination of iron and folic acid for use during pregnancy is called Pregaday.

The background cacophony of drug names helps the process of promotion. Give your detailman an easy-association name to roll readily off his tongue and onto the prescription pad, and you are home and dry. Crowded and confused lists aid this process in that the physician will accept the promoted names and differentiate in their favour for his own safety. The demonstration that high prescribers show greater brand loyalty than their more moderate brethren[23] confirms this. When confronted by Labiton, Labophyline, Laborprin or Labosept, or, say, Metamucil, Metanium or Metatone, and five minutes for the average consultation, diagnosis and prescription, the loudest and most persistent source of clarity will be relied upon.

Our last executive game has its roots in the medicinal past. It is 'This AND That'. The medicine showman, peddling his usually alcoholic medicine from the tailgate of his wagon, would, during his entertaining sales spiel, run his eye sharply over his audience. 'Unrivalled for aches, pains, boils, warts, bruises, AND spots on the nose!' An example of a modern 'AND That' is Valium. At first it was offered for relieving anxiety AND relaxing muscles. AND epilepsy, AND cardiovascular problems. Eventually it was recommended for back troubles AND apparently anything else. This is known as 'Spread of Indications'.

As part of overall marketing strategy a large multinational corporation will frequently spawn several local subsidiaries, or associate companies, in each country in which it operates. This gives a wider representation and allows more possible moves on the marketing chess board. At this corporate level further obvious strategies have been observed.

'Peter and Paul', or 'Mutt and Jeff', are brothers who work under the close direction of their father. Peter has a product that has been doing well, but eventually sales begin to fall. Enter brother Paul with essentially the same product, but with a new name, a new package and perhaps a slightly different molecule, which is promoted as obviously better. Eventually Paul takes over Peter's market, and with all the fuss probably extends it. Exit brothers smiling to praise from happy father.

A very common corporate game is 'Me-Too', and its results are naturally enough known as 'Me-Too-ers'. When knowledge of a successful formulation becomes generally available, other companies may decide to produce a similar drug to take a share of the market. (This itself may be a Peter and Paul ploy.) The drugs they produce, while not identical, will be similar enough to have the same therapeutic use and yet qualify for their own patents. Me-Too drugs are commonplace; among the hypnotics for example, nitrazepam, flurazepam and triazolam (Mogadon, Dalmane and Halcion) are effectively interchangeable. The rationale for this game is, 'If he can make a profit from it, why not me too?' Why not indeed?

The nastiest game is to sell someone your rotten fish. Many companies play this game, and the rules are fixed by the least scrupulous. It goes like this. A drug, or a group of similar drugs, is widely prescribed in the richer countries. Time and experience show that such serious and frequent adverse reactions are produced that regulatory bodies pronounce limitations or bans upon the drug's use. Unfortunately the producers have large stocks of the drug, a lot of time and money have been invested in its development, and a process is running which is constantly churning out more. What can be done with these unwanted and dangerous drugs?

The answer is simple. These drugs can be exported to poorer countries where there may be less regulation on their use,[24] the doctors are more naive, and the companies have a much higher number of detailmen to boost sales.[25]

There are many examples of this game in operation. Chloramphenicol, a potent but dangerous antibiotic, has been calculated to have caused more than 10,000 deaths from aplastic anaemia in Japan. Despite warnings to doctors about the risks, sales increased year by year until strict limitations on its use were introduced in 1975. Exports of chloramphenicol from Japan to Asian countries, especially Taiwan, rose sharply just after these restrictions came into force.[26]

The Japanese have found themselves on the receiving end of the rotten fish game. Clioquinol was developed as a germicide by Ciba-Geigy in 1899. In the 1930s they began to sell it as an anti-diarrhoeal agent, and it was accepted in Japan as 'Seichozai', which means a stomach-preparing drug.

In the United States in 1960 the FDA drastically restricted the indications for the use of clioquinol. Simultaneously Ciba-Geigy increased their marketing effort in Japan. The drug causes a distinctive syndrome, SMON (subacute myelo-optico-neuropathy), characterised by irreversible symptoms which include abnormal sensations in the lower half of the body, pain, convulsions, severe chill, paralysis and eye problems. The number of SMON victims increased rapidly in Japan in the 1960s until the Health and Welfare Ministry banned clioquinol in 1970. Ciba-Geigy was still selling the drug in those countries which permitted it in 1980, but its main markets are now in the developing countries.[27]

Lest this game should seem to be a Japanese peculiarity, examples can be found involving North American – and European-based drug manufacturers and their relationships with most third world countries. Even the most respected companies send their unwanted drugs to poor countries. ICI, now the fifth largest chemical business in the world, gave supplies of Eraldin (practolol) to the KCMC hospital in Moshi, Tanzania, in 1976, after the drug had been withdrawn from the British market because of its horrific effects.[28]

The widespread practice of neglecting to provide adequate information on drug hazards compounds the risks while making this sort of activity even more commercially attractive, as does the exaggeration of the range of use indications for the products. Milton Silverman's documentation of this situation[29] has led to some reduction in its prevalence in Latin America, but grossly exaggerated claims combined with minimal warnings are still all too common throughout the less regulated markets as our comparison of MIMS Africa and MIMS UK shows.

In reply to such criticism the industry has a well-worn selection of defences.[30] The most prominent and effective is 'We are not breaking any laws.' The companies involved insist that their foreign operations are directed by nationals of the countries concerned, who are familiar with the local laws and regulations, and who abide by them. This seemed to be an airtight defence in early United States Senate hearings and meetings of worried stockholders. However, California newspaper publisher Edgar Elfstrom and Dr Silverman were able to demonstrate that some companies had been less than frank in offering this excuse.

If their moral precepts are questioned the industry tends to reply, 'Well, things are different in Latin America.' Perhaps this attitude relies on the assumption that life is cheaper in third world countries. After all, 'it's accepted business practice,' one Latin American drug promotion expert explained; if your competitor claims five indications for his product you should claim at least six. And if he discloses three adverse reactions, you are mad if you disclose more than two.

The companies have been known to claim that 'the discrepancies in drug promotion are merely honest differences in opinion.' An anonymous Colombian health official, quoted by Dr Silverman, commented: 'When we find the company tells one story in Bogota, another in Brasilia, another in Guatemala City, and still another in Mexico City, that is difficult to comprehend.'

Experience has taught corporations that there are two games it is better not to play: price-cutting and patent-busting. When penicillin was made available to various manufacturers at the end of the Second World War, the price for a million units fell from $200 to $60 over eight years. The folly of this was underlined when it was realised that prices as such did not affect the market. It was probably the last price free-for-all that the industry suffered. The solution was to get patent protection, and the anti-biotic race was on.

There were three winners of the commercial race. Parke Davis applied for a patent for chloramphenicol in October 1949, Cyanamid applied with chlortetracycline in September 1949 and Pfizer with oxytetracycline in July 1950. During the next two years Pfizer noticed tetracycline within oxytetracycline and chlortetracycline, and they produced it. They applied for a patent in October 1952, and rival claims for the same compound rapidly followed from Cyanamid and Bristol. In January 1955 Pfizer convinced the United States Patents Office that they should be granted the patent for tetracycline.

From there we fall into 'an antibiotic broth spiced with the laws of patents and unfair methods of competition'[31] in the shape of a US Federal Trade Commission Report. To which are devoted 11,000 pages of record, 8,000 pages of exhibits, many thousands of pages of briefs and two days of good appeal argument, all 'In the matter of American Cyanamid Co., Bristol-Myers Co., Bristol Laboratories Inc., Chas Pfizer and Co. Inc., Olin Mathieson Chemical Corporation (Squibb) and the Upjohn Co.'

It emerged that Pfizer had managed to convince the Patents Officer that the chemical structure of chlortetracycline and oxytetracycline had not been known to them at the time that tetracycline had been discovered through the screening of over 100,000 soil samples. There was no question of copying; it was a genuine discovery. While the decision on Pfizer's application was pending, an adaptive corporate response had started. Together with Cyanamid, Pfizer planned an 'amicable settlement' in advance of the outcome. This involved a cross-licensing agreement, so that there would be no losers.

Things settled down comfortably until 1961, when it was alleged in a complaint to the Kefauver Commission that 'Pfizer had made false, mis-leading and incorrect statements for the purpose of inducing the US Patents Office to grant a patent on tetracycline'. In short, a plot was described, in which Pfizer, Cyanamid and Bristol had all witheld information from the Patents Officer. It was concluded that the Pfizer/ Cyanamid control of the tetracycline market was based on misrepresentation and distastefully unclean hands. They had not played the game according to the legal rules. No matter, they carried on as if nothing had happened, using their patent rights to defend both market and price,[32] although knowledge of this may have prompted the action taken by the British Minister of Health and ICI to break the Pfizer hold on the British tetracycline market.

The Kefauver anti-trust hearings exposed much of the inner workings of the industry to the outside world. Additionally the hearings were expensive, time consuming and generally undesirable. It would obviously make better sense for the companies to conduct themselves in ways which would not lead to intervention in their affairs by the authorities. This seemed to be the case until 1979 when an antibiotic once more led to the institution of an anti-trust suit against Eli Lilly in the cephalosporin market.[33]

The drugs and marketing manoeuvres we have been discussing are concerned with established areas of medication and the drugs that compete to service them. But what of forward market areas? The boards of directors of Japanese industrial corporations are reported to be concerned actively with defining markets for their products twenty years hence. Are drug companies any different? They do have one theoretical problem that does not confront conventional industry: how is the pharmaceutical industry to maintain profits and growth in the future given that there is a finite amount of disease in the world, which should, if its efforts are effective, actually be decreasing?

The direction the drug manufacturers have chosen to pursue is the unlimited area of human variability. Within human variability they have identified conditions and situations which have then been generalised and declared suitable for treatment. Inevitably this involves grey areas of indistinct or dubious medical judgement, where the application of pressure can easily persuade in favour of treatment with drugs. Problems of the human condition become medical problems. Social and emotional situations of everyday life become diseases treatable with drugs, and in the process symptoms are elevated to the status of serious diseases.

Perhaps the most disturbing human generalisation involves the abuse of children with behaviour-modifying stimulant drugs. This practice was first exposed in America by Robert Maynard in the *Washington Post* in 1970,[34] but it has its roots in work undertaken in the early 1960s. Ciba first proposed that their amphetamine-like drug Ritalin (methylphenidate) should be used for children in 1961, as a treatment for functional behaviour problems. This approach was rebuffed by the FDA, but by 1963 the company had gained approval for this use of the drug.[35] In the same year the US Public Health Services and the National Society for Crippled Children and Adults sponsored a seminar on the 'Child with Minimal Brain Dysfunction (MBD)'. A task force was formed from this seminar to identify and label this previously unrecognised type of child.

By 1966 a definition, of sorts, of children suffering from MBD had been produced. They turn out to be 'children of near average, average, or above average general intelligence with certain learning or behavioural disabilities ranging from mild to severe, which are associated with deviations of function of the central nervous system. These deviations may manifest themselves by various combinations of impairment in perception, conceptualization, language, memory and control of attention, impulse or motor function.'[36] To clarify any doubt that may remain in identifying MBD a further ninety-nine symptoms are listed. They include: hyper and hypo (too much and too little) activity, rage and tantrum reactions, being sweet and even-tempered, being cooperative and friendly, being gullible and easily led, being socially bold and aggressive, being sensitive to others, being a light sleeper, or being a heavy sleeper. In fact just being seems to be sufficient to qualify any child for diagnosis as suffering from MBD.

The groundwork of the task force was further consolidated when its head, Dr S. Clements, subsequently worked as a consultant for Ciba-Geigy and produced their physicians' handbook on MBD. By 1975 around one million US children were diagnosed as suffering from MBD. Of these, 515,000 were treated with drugs; 265,000 were given Ritalin.[37]

But what exactly is MBD? Its key concept appears to be that of hyperactivity (hyperkinesis). Some, indeed it might be argued all, children are at times over-active and do not pay attention in school. They may also be clumsy, have learning or speech difficulties and act impulsively. Under pressure doctors have been persuaded to diagnose this behaviour as a medical condition, for which a suitably impressive name has been used. In minimal brain dysfunction, how minimal is minimal? Since so little is actually known about the normal functioning of the brain, fine graduations of dysfunction clearly provide a very fertile grey area in which to promote a disease. It is extremely rare that clear evidence of brain damage can be found in MBD cases. And as any parent will have deduced from the symptoms, it is difficult to tell a normally restless or rebellious child from one that might be said to have MBD. There are no laboratory tests or definitive examinations for MBD; it has in fact become a popular catch-all diagnosis for children who misbehave in school or have learning problems.[38]

It would appear that in America, where youth is simultaneously envied and resented, the drug manufacturers have found a suitable schism in which they may spread both disease and cure. Such widespread drugging of children cannot be attributed to the carelessness of the odd individual physician. It is a product of the combined forces of several institutions within that society: the drug industry, the educational system, the medical profession, and not least a result of the way parents have been conditioned to view their children.

Against this background, Ciba-Geigy are able to estimate that one in twenty children have MBD. Some parents will take heart in the report that 'these drugs bring about amazing results within ten minutes after ingestion, making the child calm, attentive, and co-operative'.[39] Observers who have labelled the history of the marketing of Ritalin 'a cure in search of a disease',[40] however, draw support from those parents who have noticed that the 'symptoms' of MBD miraculously abate during school vacations.

Essentially we must ask, are children being abused and controlled with drugs simply because school is boring?

The headache is an example of an everyday problem which was elevated to a disease. Everyone suffers the occasional headache; it is usually a minor symptom that something needs changing. Fresh air, something to eat or drink, perhaps a little exercise, might be all the body requires to eliminate the symptom, or at most a mild analgesic such as aspirin or paracetamol. But when almost every headache comes to be called a 'migraine', and the condition is widely reputed to be a common affliction of the more intelligent and successful, then migraine becomes a fashionable disease requiring a doctor's attention and prescribed drugs. Initially the drug of choice was ergotamine tartrate, which can prevent migraine, but if it is used over long periods it can also induce it. So this fashion actually led to an increase in genuine migraine, through the sufferers of ergotamine-induced migraine.[41] More recently a range of drugs has been developed for perpetual use by migraine sufferers. They are intended to prevent attacks; they certainly raise chronic drug use to a level which is likely to continue, even in the absence of the disease it is intended to treat.

Bed-wetting is another transient human condition. And although with some kids it can appear to go on forever, most are dry by the age of five, but around 10 per cent can still be expected to wet the bed occasionally. Even at ten years old perhaps 5 per cent will still do it now and then. It is all part of the processes of growing and adjusting, and by seven or eight years persistent bed-wetters begin to worry about it and usually stop.[42] For parents it can be a nuisance, but it requires a distorted perspective to regard it as an illness.

But bed-wetting has been given the name enuresis and made into a treatable condition. The drugs used are imipramine, marketed as Tofranil by Geigy, and amitriptyline, marketed as Tryptizol by Merck, Sharp & Dohme. They seldom have the desired effect on the under eights, and the over eights adjust themselves. Apart from their apparent pointlessness, these drugs are particularly poisonous, and have been prescribed so freely that in Britain they were the commonest form of fatal poisoning in children under the age of five years in the late 1970s.

Geigy produced imipramine as Tofranil syrup. Syrup is a common way of making medicines palatable to young patients; tragically, it can make them popular to the point of easy overdose. The *British Medical Journal* published a harrowing case history under the title 'Poisoning with tricyclic antidepressants: an avoidable cause of childhood death'.[43] They reported:

> A four year old boy weighing 14 kg (31 lbs) drank 90 ml of Tofranil syrup which had been prescribed for his bedwetting. His mother, who was unaware of the poisonous nature of the drug, gave him a salt and water mixture, after which he vomited and then went to sleep. Four hours later he had a generalised fit, which lasted until he was given intravenous diazepam (Valium) in hospital. After this he remained unconscious but responded to painful stimuli. The electrocardiograph showed sinus rhythm with a rate of 180/minute; his blood pressure was 110/70. Shortly after admission he developed ventricular tachycardia. Intravenous physostigmine and lignocaine failed to control this but after disopryamide, 25 mg given intravenously, sinus rhythm was restored. Cardiac monitoring was continued and he remained in sinus rhythm with a heart rate of 160–180/minute until 18 hours after ingestion of the drug when he developed ventricular fibrillation. Sinus rhythm and an adequate circulation were restored by DC countershock but he had a further episode of ventricular fibrillation two hours later and could not be resuscitated.

This sweet syrup had caused a small boy to go into continuous convulsions which could be suppressed only with another drug. Later, his heart began to malfunction so seriously that he eventually died. The *BMJ* leader in the same issue[44] comments: 'There is no specific antidote, and treatment of massive overdosage is difficult. These effects have been well reported but there seems to be widespread ignorance of the lethal nature of the drug.'

Need our common sense desert us, with such disastrous consequences? Would it matter if this small boy, and the many others who have suffered the same horrible fate, wet their beds for years? It is fortunate that the promotion of human conditions into diseases to be treated with drugs does not always have such deadly conclusions.

In lighter vein, an example of condition medicine has been provided by Zyma (UK) Ltd, an associate of Geigy. Studying pharmaceutical advertising in the medical press, we found it hard to resist their campaign for Paroven. This is a drug which causes blood vessels near the surface of the body to dilate; it can be prescribed for haemorrhoids or venous insufficiency. The campaign centres around a pair of beautiful, healthy young legs, lying down, standing up and bound in various ways with red and blue ropes. There are even posters featuring these lovely naked legs: not for the consulting room obviously, but they arrive in the doctor's mail. The word scan varies; this month's special feature is 'cramps', other symptoms of the month include 'heavy legs', 'painful legs', and – our choice every time – 'restless legs'. To keep this horrendous affliction at bay, it is suggested that initially you require three or four Paroven a day, and then a maintenance dose of one a day.[45] For life.

Situation medicine is essentially medicine for every occasion. In promoting situation medicine the art is to find a common situation which is generally disliked in everyday life. All experiences in our lives bring biological responses, some of which we judge pleasant, and others unpleasant. They all have some meaning, and in suppressing or modifying them without regard to their content, we may simply be increasing the possibility of serious damage and disease at a later date.

The success of promotion campaigns for situation medicines hinge predominantly on questions of perception. And behind perception lies the cultural, ethnic or moral basis of our relationship with the society of which we are a part. The assumptions of this relationship are the springboards of drug promotion. To illustrate crudely, if a celibate priest were to wake and find himself to have been divinely transported to the middle of a crowded nudist beach in mid-summer, his response to the situation might lead a doctor to diagnose extreme anxiety, hypertension and perhaps acute respiratory problems. To the majority of bathers the situation would be one of healthy relaxation or beneficial exercise. Only their perception of it would differ.

Physicians, at whom these campaigns are aimed, are not qualified to make judgements of the type involved in prescribing drugs to change perception. Questions about behaviour, education, morality and the boundaries of 'normality' inevitably arise, and any answer must be arbitary and therefore unsatisfactory. Many physicians accept this, but under pressure from patients and the pharmaceutical industry, and in the absence of any mechanism for the solution of such highly individual problems, they have little option but to prescribe.

The Rolling Stones' 'Mother's Little Helpers' was both a reflection and an overture to what was to become the most common area of promotional drama: the housewife, suffering from her life situation. One advertisement shows a young, attractive, affluent woman with clean children and material goods and other symbols of the things that are considered desirable and necessary to her. But acute anxiety and emotional turmoil seethe beneath the chic exterior. The cause of this lamentable state of affairs may well be her apparent total inability to choose decisively one of the eight brands of breakfast cereal on offer to her. One ad of this type is captioned 'Now she can cope'. She has taken Stelazine to help her through the maze of the supermarket. 'Stelazine: the one to turn to . . . when she's suffering from anxiety and finds it difficult to cope.'

Smith, Kline & French produce Stelazine (trifluoperazine hydrochloride). It is one of the major tranquillizers, a drug which can be used to treat the most severe type of mental illness, schizophrenia, as well as labyrinthine disorders. We have all experienced the labyrinth problem of finding what we want in the supermarket, and no doubt felt near the brink of schizophrenia when confronted by a multiplicity of breakfast cereals; but is this tenuous connection sufficient to justify persuading the medical profession to prescribe powerful anti-psychotic drugs to harrassed housewives?

The Stelazine advertisement claims that it brings 'relief . . . usually without problems of dependence'. Valium, the market leader among the minor tranquillizers, is advertised, except in America, without mention of dependence, or addiction as it is less politely called. Originally tranquillizers of this sort were believed to be without addiction problems, but in recent years the true nature of the dependence has emerged,[46] and in some parts of the United States there are now 'Pills Anonymous' groups attempting to cope with the victims. Current adverts for the drug do not mention addiction as one of the hazards, but tell how 'day-to-day stressors of living – . . . marriage . . . singlehood . . . income and employment . . . finance . . . – can lead to *disabling* tension and anxiety.' (Our emphasis) It continues: 'Current life stressors are amenable to correction through relevant treatment programs . . . Valium (diazepam/Roche) may be your best pharmacologic measure to relieve excessive anxiety – Valium when anxiety is greater than the patient's ability to cope.'

Jill McDougall is a housewife who knows the consequence of such ready use of Valium. She just phones her doctor's receptionist to get prescriptions for 100 tablets as often as she wants, because nobody takes her seriously, or wants to listen to her long enough to find out what is really wrong. The psychiatrist who first gave her Valium said 'You won't get hooked. What do you think you are, a hippy or something?' Now Jill can't stop taking them; without them her stomach becomes tight and painful and she is overtaken by totally disabling panic. 'You really need them,' she explained. She was horrified to find herself a drug addict, but she is one of thousands, possibly millions, in the same situation throughout the world. The stress induced by the withdrawal of Valium is, in the words of the advert, 'greater than the patient's ability to cope'.

Living in high-rise housing is sufficient reason for a woman to need antidepressants, according to a Triptafen advertisement. The indication for the use of the antidepressant Prothiaden is distress in yet another supermarket, choosing toilet rolls this time. Tranxene is promoted for the inherent stress of studenthood, especially for the girls because of their 'natural desire to be feminine'. Housework is the context for the need for Limbritol, while the working wife and mother suffers 'a deep feeling of guilt, a feeling which persists despite the activities of women's lib'. For women, allegedly every life situation can lead to an unavoidable dependence upon psychotropic drugs.

Condition and situation medicine illustrate the growth of practices which, if not challenged and checked, could progressively classify all natural physical and emotional responses as medical conditions requiring drug therapy. The responses of our bodies and minds to work, environmental or life situations have developed throughout our evolution to tell us something, perhaps vital, about what is happening to us. These messages and the feelings and reactions they produce are the essence of an animate being. It seems stupid in the extreme to blot them out, to cancel their effects with increasing doses of drugs. Although when an estimated 100 million more-or-less willing victims take tranquillizers every day in the Western world,[47] it may not be surprising that we are so complacent about this issue.

Even when an easily corrected lifestyle problem is acknowledged by the pharmaceutical industry and medical profession alike to be the prime cause of symptoms, drugs are promoted as suitable treatment. In Britain and the United States the problems associated with an over-refined diet are made particularly acute by the universal availability of the disgusting white sliced loaf. A diet lacking sufficient natural fibre can cause constipation, which, if persistent can lead to diverticular disease, inflamed lesions in the muscular bowel wall.[48] This may cause the bowel to cease to function adequately and the eventual result can be fatal bowel cancer. It would seem relatively easy for doctors to give simple dietary advice to their patients so that they may avoid the trail of woe that an unsuitable diet can bring: vegetables, grains and fruits in due proportion, processed as little as possible. Of course, there is another way. A Reckitt and Coleman advertisement shows a blue-haired lady daintily holding a white, crust-free sandwich to her lips. 'Dorothy's refined habits,' the caption reads, 'have led to a serious problem.' Doctors are advised to prescribe Fybogel sachets containing ispaghula husk BPC, 'the natural way to end dietary constipation'.

The long-term mis-match between lifestyles and our bodies' needs often causes problems which become apparent only after many years. As we age, the components and systems degenerate, particularly if they are mis-used, and the resulting symptoms can sometimes be relieved by drugs. The problem lies in selecting the best course of action to take when there are signs of a developing malfunction. Some types of intervention may cause more problems than they solve. These are clearly matters for debate, where opinion can take precedence over fact.

The treatment of high blood pressure is a good example of such a controversial area. Over the past decade there has been an intense campaign for mass detection and medication of hypertensives – individuals whose blood pressure is considered to be dangerously high. With the launch of yet another new antihypertensive drug in Britain in May 1981, clinical pharmacologist Professor Paul Turner of St Bartholomew's was reported in a major daily newspaper to have said that 35 per cent of middle-aged adults 'suffer from above-average' blood pressure, and are therefore at risk of early death.[49] Remarks such as these do not escape the attention of the pharmaceutical industry as however you define the average, this is potentially an enormous lucrative market.

We shall deal with hypertension in some detail because it provides an excellent example of pharmaceutical industry strategy.

Blood is pumped around the body under pressure by the heart. In normal people, blood pressure varies about an average figure at different times of the day and with different circumstances. In the developed world, blood pressure has been found to rise with increasing age. Blood pressure measurement produces two figures. The first – it may be about 120 mm Hg in a normal person – is the pressure at which the blood is pumped out of the heart; and the second, which varies around 80 mm Hg, is the resting pressure between pulses when the heart is filling up ready for the next squeeze. They are known as systolic and diastolic pressures respectively, and written like this: 120/80.

High blood pressure is important because it is statistically associated with reduced life expectancy and serious illness. It can lead to a failure of the fine blood vessels in susceptible organs such as the kidneys, eyes and brain through simple mechanical damage. Naturally, insurance companies are interested in these effects, and diagram 3 shows how the blood pressure figures are used to build up a probability figure for life expectancy. The higher up the steps your blood pressure puts you, the more serious will be the reaction of your doctor and insurance company.

Hypertension is an ideal case for mass medication because it is very difficult to make a decision about the cut-off point between hypertension and acceptable blood pressure. It is a classic grey area. With a continuous variable of this sort, there can be no clear-cut level about which different people will be in unequivocal agreement.[50] It is the subject of regular and lengthy debate in the medical journals, and serious proposals are made frequently for drug treatment of that large proportion of the population which might be at risk.[51] Physicians are under considerable pressure to intervene, especially from the drug manufacturers, who subject them to a constant barrage of promotional material, drawing on the published debate for much of their ammunition. But to attempt to keep blood pressure down through indefinite medication, without attempting to deal with its causes, is like trying to cool a room by chilling the thermometer.

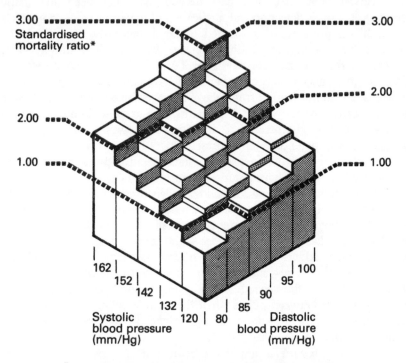

3.00   Standardised mortality ratio*

* STANDARDISED MORTALITY RATIO is the ratio of the mortality rate for a particular subgroup to the mortality rate for the population at large, standardised for age and sex. So, according to the diagram, people with diastolic blood pressure of 100 and systolic pressure of 162 are three times more likely to die than others of the same age and sex, on average.

Diagram 3. Adapted from Society of Actuaries Build and Blood Pressure Study 1959 and relates to men aged 40–69.

The body's answer to many assaults of modern living – smoking, high salt diet, sedentary lifestyle and certain commonly used drugs – is an increase in blood pressure. It seems to be an incidental effect of a natural mechanism that animals use to numb themselves against stress or pain. Stimulation of pressure receptors in the blood vessels and heart reduces fear, and it seems likely that hypertension helps chronically stressed people to cope.[52]

As long ago as 1908, it was thought that 'hurry, worry and angry emotions had much to do with hypertension in man'.[53] It can, for example, result from stress due to overcrowding. In prisons hypertension is more common than outside, and its incidence shows a direct linear relationship with the number of square feet available to each inmate.[54]

In most cases, blood pressure falls when stress levels fall. For many hypertensives, a simple sleeping and resting regimen designed to prevent chronic exhaustion is enough to prevent the condition from recurring. Consultant cardiologist Dr Peter Nixon, who treats hypertensives with problems serious enough to involve the heart, finds that counselling on the management of the condition is sufficient treatment for the majority. 'Fewer than ten per cent,' he reports, 'appear to have secondary hypertension or a permanently established condition requiring drug therapy.'[55]

Even such limited measures as weight loss and reduction of sodium intake can be remarkably effective, allowing at least 85 per cent of borderline hypertensives to achieve normal blood pressure. Excessive dietary sodium – in salt and food additives such as monosodium glutamate and baking powder – may be the major cause of the epidemic of hypertension in 'civilised' countries,[56] for not only do we add salt to our food but we consume large quantities of high-sodium processed foods ranging from Kelloggs Corn Flakes (260 mg per ounce) to hamburgers (1510 mg in Macdonald's 'Big Mac').[57] The calorie content of these foods adds to the problem: hypertension is twice as common among overweight people as among the underweight,[58] and one study showed that an average fall in blood pressure of 16.7/8.4 mm Hg accompanies a weight loss of 3 kg (about 7 lb) or more.[59]

Such approaches hold no appeal for the pharmaceutical industry. Nor, apparently, for many members of the medical profession. The medical approach is typified by the Tufts-New England Medical Center Family Health Guide, *What You Can Do About High Blood Pressure*.[60] Introducing the subject of treatment, it asserts: 'Except for the small number of people for whom the cause of hypertension can be eliminated (the 'secondary' hypertensives), the disease has to be brought and kept under control through the use of drugs . . . *Treatment of hypertension is a life-long undertaking* . . . Protection from the hazards of hypertension lasts only as long as the medication is taken as directed.'

The antihypertensive campaign has been through a sequence of phases. Early advertisements concentrated on alerting doctors to the importance of hypertension and proposed that they check their patients' blood pressure more often than hitherto. High blood pressure, a symptom of underlying problems, which often causes the patient no discomfort, was subtly elevated to the status of a disease requiring medication.

In 1974, Merck, Sharp & Dohme were advising physicians that 10 per cent of their patients could be undiscovered hypertensives. A typical advertisement showed a worker who had 'had a bit of an accident', and the text, reminding the doctor that 'two extra minutes of your time could add years to his life', advised that 'No doctor should miss an opportunity to record the blood pressure of a young or middle-aged patient who is a rare visitor to the surgery.' If hypertension is revealed, Aldomet (methyldopa) should be prescribed.

Casual blood pressure measurement represents a sound strategy for the drug companies. By this means at any particular time, about 20 per cent of the population can be classified as hypertensive, but repeated measurements show that more than half of those initially believed to be hypertensive in fact have fluctuating blood pressure, or labile hypertension.[61] Writing in the *Journal of the American Medical Association*, Dr Irvine Page warned that 'many subjects receive a misdiagnosis by careless screening, especially the millions of borderline hypertensive persons. It is wicked to label a person hypertensive only because one or two measurements show mild systolic hypertension. This may mean a lifetime of taking a drug in useless quantities and a lifetime of anxiety.'[62]

Anxiety is crucial to the success of the antihypertensive campaign. Fear of the possible consequences of neglecting to treat hypertension is the goad which drives doctors to prescribe and which they in turn use to ensure their patients' compliance in taking the pills. This essentially negative approach characterises the industry-sponsored literature.

Smith, Kline & French provide an example of 'education' about hypertension which would tend to induce anxiety. It is an expensively produced 'learning program' forming a series of six units on 'Risk Management of the Hypertensive Patient'. Under the august chairmanship of Alfred Soffer MD, Executive Director of the American College of Chest Physicians, Editor-in-Chief of *Chest* and Editor of *Archives of Internal Medicine*, the direction and content was provided by an international committee of senior clinicians. Few doctors anywhere in the world would discount such a prestigious group.

The information given in the programme is accurate. More interesting to the discerning reader, however, is the way it is presented. The message is cumulative: 'Hypertension is a major, worldwide health problem – a typically asymptomatic disease that frequently leads to cardiovascular disease and death . . . Hypertension may affect 15 to 20 per cent of all adults.' Back-up is provided in the form of a graph giving a diastolic pressure of 95 mm Hg as the level at which hypertension should be diagnosed. The implication is that 15 to 20 per cent of the population risk death from cardiovascular disease unless constantly treated with drugs. The message is further emphasised by a warning: 'The first symptom of cardiovascular disease is often sudden death. . . .'

Scientific data showing the beneficial effects of reducing blood pressure are reported to be 'accumulating rapidly'. Significantly, the discussion of these data omits the point that none of the work reviewed shows any benefit whatever due to drug treatment for mild hypertension. This fact is in the booklet, but the reader has to make a determined effort to find it. It is in the text under a diagram for which, unfortunately in such an expensive publication, the caption is divided between two pages, thus: 'The Veterans Administrative Co-operative Study Group in the United States showed that treatment lowers blood pressure and greatly improves life expectancy'. To find the rest of the explanation, where it is admitted that the patients for whom this was true had initial diastolic pressure above 115, you have to turn to another page.

The learning programme concludes that 'Prevention – the only answer – requires early detection of highly vulnerable persons and control of the manageable predisposing factors'. Known causes of cardiovascular disease are discounted, except for cigarettes, and physicians are specifically warned that 'treatment diets may be harmful'. The reader is led to believe that the only possible way to exert 'control of the manageable predisposing factors' is through the use of drugs.

A chain of reasoning is presented that is simply not logical. But it could lead the uncritical doctor, worried about the prospect of his patients' sudden deaths, to initiate antihypertensive drug regimes with one-fifth of his patients.

The medication process can easily become progressive. If the first drug does not have the desired effect, the doctor may add others to achieve a greater reduction in blood pressure. Many patients end up taking beta-blockers, diuretics and tranquillizers, or methyldopa and a selection of the others. With many diuretics, potassium supplements are required; and further drug treatment may be initiated for gout or diabetes precipitated by antihypertensive therapy. And unfortunately, antihypertensive drugs can cause impotence. There is little the doctor can do about this, but it is predictable that the marital problems that follow may lead to stress, hypertension and more pills.

The effectiveness of the antihypertensive campaign can be seen in prescribing figures for Britain. Over a decade, the rise in the number of prescriptions for antihypertensive drugs has outstripped all others except the tranquillizers – which are themselves often used as part of the treatment regime for high blood pressure. From 1966 to 1975, diuretic prescribing trebled while tranquillizers doubled and specific drugs acting on the heart (including beta-blockers) increased by three-quarters. In cost terms, the NHS bill for antihypertensive drugs rose from £6 million to £20 million, for diuretics from £4 million to £20 million, for heart preparations, from £1 million to £17 million, and for tranquillizers from £6 million to £13 million.[63] Some of the additional cost can be accounted for in terms of the development of increasingly expensive drugs, particularly beta-blockers, but there has also been a massive increase in the volume of drugs prescribed.

A similar massive surge in antihypertensive medication has also occurred in other parts of the world. In the United States in 1980, the five leading drugs included only one, an analgesic, which could not be prescribed specifically for hypertension. Of the other four, one was a beta-blocker (Inderal), two were diuretics (Dyazide and Lasix) and the fourth was Valium.[64] Among Sweden's top five were two different beta-blockers and two diuretics.[65] In Norway prescribing of antihypertensive drugs more than doubled between 1971 and 1977, and beta-blockers in particular are still rising fast.[66] The pharmaceutical industry still considers hypertension to be the most important worldwide area for expansion.

In Britain the Blood Pressure Boom has brought drug companies increased sales revenue of about £180 million over a ten-year period. In the United States the market was worth an estimated $1,400 million in 1981,[67] with a projected annual rate of growth of 10 to 15 per cent. For beta-blockers, the growth rate forecast is nearer 30 per cent.[68]

One would expect the bogey of heart disease to be in retreat, if not stopped in its tracks by this explosion of attention and expenditure. Yet in Britain in 1979 deaths from heart disease reached new record levels.[69] But this is not true of the United States, where heart disease has begun to decline. This is very interesting, since medication strategies are similar on both sides of the Atlantic, and the more affluent Americans tend to have a less suitable diet than the British. So why the difference? The answer seems to lie in two factors outside the scope of medication. First, in the hundreds of millions of dollars that have been spent on public education on smoking, diet and exercise, augmented by the more precise food labelling required in the United States. The second is in the application of this education; the growing American passion for fitness, reflected in an estimated twenty-five million joggers, is unparalleled in Britain. The British seem more content to rely on their National Health Service, which in turn relies predominantly on drugs.

What will be the next commercial focus of the drug manufacturers? The 1950s saw the antibiotic boom; psychotropics flowered in the 1960s; antihypertensives dominated the 1970s. For the 1980s 'a highly dynamic growth period' is forecast for antidiabetic drugs. A major market research report on the pharmaceutical industry published in March 1981 said: 'Diabetes may become a new "in" disease in the 1980s, just as hypertension and cancer are now'. United States sales of antidiabetic drugs are expected to rise from $222 million in 1980 to $775 million in 1988.[70]

Shall we see in this decade a campaign for the detection and treatment of millions of previously undiscovered diabetics? Diabetes has all the characteristics of a grey area disease; it is associated with seriously reduced life expectancy; it is the most common single cause of blindness; it is associated with serious cardiovascular problems. That highly potent motivator, fear of early death or disability, can be readily invoked. Detection, by a simple urine test, is quick and can be carried out in the doctor's surgery or the patient's home.

The enterprising Germans have already made a significant start. Euglucon 5 (glibenclamide) manufactured by Boehr M/Hoechst, was the best-selling drug in West Germany from mid-1980 to mid-1981. The sales value of this antidiabetic was DM300 million ($20 million), compared to DM180 million of its nearest rival Tagamet (cimetidine) during this period.[71]

It is clearly worthwhile, if not essential, for drug companies to emphasise the creation of disease, and to encourage doctors to seek out such illnesses and provide long-term drug treatment, regardless of any question of genuine benefit to patients.

Every part of our bodies, every response to mental and physical stimulation, and every conceivable social interaction have become legitimate prey for the business strategy of the drug manufacturers. There is a continuous search, not for disease or disability that may be cured or aided, but for conditions that may be profitably promoted for drug treatment. Ultimately the result of these strategies must be iatrogenic disease.

The success of the strategies of the drug manufacturers are obvious. In Britain some statistics[72] on drug costs and prescribing are published by the Department of Health and Social Security (DHSS), the department which pays for the NHS, and consequently for the vast majority of all drugs prescribed in the country. Since the Health Service began in 1948 the drug bill has risen every year. Initially it was a fairly slow rise, around £5 million each year. But through the decade of the 1970s the rate of growth of the drug bill accelerated to reach a staggering £1,000 million by the end of the decade. Diagram 4 shows the drug bill for Britain. It appears to be an exponential curve, rising out of sight with horrifying speed.

In the United States total drug expenditure has also risen, as diagram 5 shows. The rate of acceleration is not as great as in Britain, perhaps because more of the direct cost comes out of the consumer's pocket.

The steeply rising drugs bill of most countries cannot be attributed to inflation or rising drug costs. Quite simply the good business sense of the pharmaceutical industry is ensuring that more and more drugs are being consumed for more and more complaints and conditions. The final diagram below shows the rise in the number of prescriptions issued in Britain. As mentioned, the middle 1960s saw the tranquillizer boom, and the 1970s were the beginning of the continuing boom in antihypertensives.

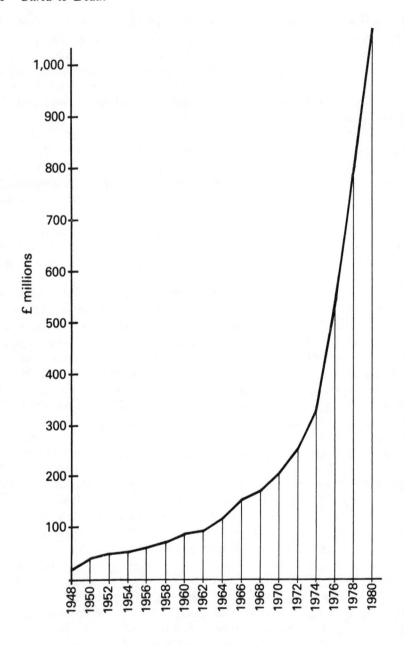

Diagram 4. Escalating cost of NHS prescriptions in Great Britain.

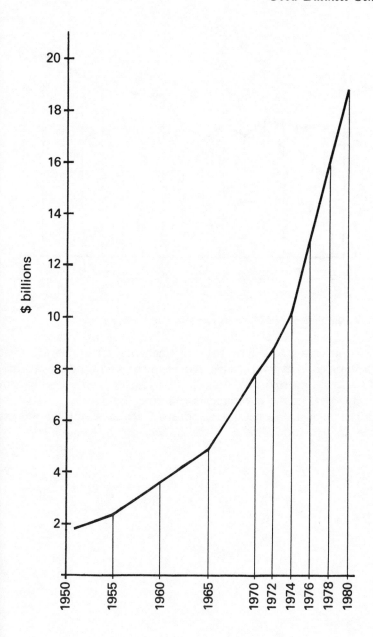

Diagram 5. Escalating value of United States Pharmaceuticals. Various sources.

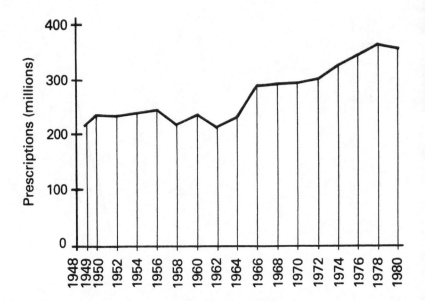

Diagram 6. Number of NHS prescriptions in Great Britain.

There is no reason to believe that the trends illustrated above are not being encouraged in every available market in the world, by the pharmaceutical industry, assisted by the medical professions, and generally with the tacit approval of the governments concerned.

The multinational pharmaceutical industries are some of the healthiest businesses in the world. But how healthy are we, their customers?

Chapter Six

Evidence and Effects

In 1828 P.C.A. Louis at the Charity Hospital, Paris, made one of the first scientific attempts to measure the value of therapy. He examined the effects of bleeding in patients with pneumonia. Louis concluded that the longer bleeding was delayed the better the outcome for the patient and he suggested that the outcome might be improved still further *if no blood was let at all*. He found that at that time in Paris the practice was so firmly established that failing to let blood in a serious illness was tantamount to gross professional negligence.

In the 1950's in the UK to fail to use anticoagulant drugs in a patient with coronary disease almost constituted negligence in the view of some doctors. *The demonstration that therapy is of no use, or even that it is harmful, does not always lead to its abandonment.*

Paul Ehrlich was very specific in 1906. 'In order to use chemotherapy successfully, we must search for substances which have an affinity for the cells of the parasite and a power of killing them *greater than the damage such substances causes to the organism itself, so that the destruction of the parasite will be possible without seriously hurting the organism.*'

– V. Coleman, *The Medicine Men*

Conventional wisdom assumes that under medical supervision drugs are beneficial. Medicines are given most of the credit for the improvements in life expectancy enjoyed by the population of the developed world. A century ago, before the development of modern drugs, death rates were undoubtedly higher in these countries than they are today. In the third world, where medical aid tends not to be readily available to the poor, enormous suffering can still be seen. But are these undeniable differences due to the use of potent drugs? Is there evidence to justify our great faith in the value of medicines? The crucial question for intensively medicated societies is, can it be proved that drugs are improving our health?

The answer to these questions can only be found through a careful examination of detailed statistics for health, illness, death and the factors which act upon them. Even in some comparatively stable countries in the developed world, accurate and complete demographic information is not always available. Whether someone is ill, or dies, may only be of interest a very few, and this is increasingly true as one moves down the economic scale amongst nations. Nevertheless, from developed countries at least, sufficient data are available from either national governments or world agencies, such as the WHO or the United Nations organisation, for some trends to be discerned.

Statistics are notoriously subject to interpretation and can produce different results in different hands. The University of Chicago produced a study which, they argued, demonstrated that use of the drug diethyl stilboestrol, a powerful synthetic oestrogen used to prevent miscarriage, caused no increase in breast cancer. Dr Sidney Wolfe, of the Public Citizen Health Research Group, reanalysed the data and came to the conclusion that among the two million women who had taken the drug, 13,000 additional cases of breast cancer could be expected. Agreeing with Wolfe's findings, Dr Gross of the FDA Bureau of Drugs said: 'I would judge these statements [by the University of Chicago] to be nothing short of nonsense.'[2]

Statistics also obscure the individual and, in the field of medicine, anomalies and exceptions are particularly common. Many of us have personal experience of lives clearly saved by the appropriate use of drugs. Every child diabetic who grows to productive adulthood is a living example of the marvel of modern medicine. Despite this, when changes in population as a whole are examined it may be found that there is a balance between the lives that are saved and the cases of drug damage and death. The problem is to determine on which side the scales are weighted. The tragedies are quietly buried, while successes are continually before us. Only a broad statistical overview can determine the reality of the situation.

Even in very limited questions of drug effects, some degree of doubt is always present. When there were already thousands of thalidomide babies all over the world, and the company which created the drug was on trial in Germany for negligence, experts were willing to testify that it could not be *proved* that thalidomide caused damage to unborn babies. For most people, however, the evidence was strong enough to convince beyond reasonable doubt.[3]

A problem inherent in almost all statistical methods is that they do not demonstrate cause-and-effect relationships. The best they can do is show associations. Thus statistical techniques could not show that thalidomide caused malformations, only that malformations were associated with the ingestion of thalidomide. In some cases where there are simple time-sequences, cause and effect can readily be distinguished, but with changes in health and drug use they are easily confused. Do I take another pill because I feel ill and it can make me well, or am I ill because I took a pill this morning? On an individual basis it might be possible to answer the question, but with whole populations it is often not.

The most reliable information about the health status of populations comes from death statistics. This is mainly because there is little ambiguity about death, and under normal circumstances it is easy to discriminate between death and life. In considering illness statistics there is much more doubt. Sociologists have made extensive studies of illness behaviour and found that one man may call himself ill and be treated as ill, and thus join the ranks of the sick, when his symptoms are much less severe than those of another. The first man may be able to afford some time being sick; he may even enjoy it; or he may want to use the time in another way. So he will be ill. Another man, however, wants to make a good impression at his new job, so he will ignore the symptoms until they disappear. He will not be ill.[4] Who is to decide which man is actually ill?

While death rates have nothing to do with individuals' perception of illness or with questions of judgement, they do have their flaws. The most serious of these is the fact that death measures only the end-point of a fatal process.[5] If we were only to look at death rates, we should miss the many non-fatal but none the less serious long-term chronic illnesses like rheumatoid arthritis. We cannot reasonably discuss the health status of a population if we ignore chronic illness, especially as this is particularly prevalent in the developed world. Nor can we ignore the number of years for which people may be disabled or crippled. Death statistics are unaffected whether death takes place after an individual has been bed-ridden and helpless for ten years, or is healthy and suddenly struck down.

In considering health our main concern should be that we stay healthy and active as long as possible, not that we suffer extended years of disabled survival. If the explosion of drug therapy has real value it should show as an increase in active life.

John and Sonja McKinlay, who have done pioneering work on this problem at Boston University, state:

> We are not merely concerned with the prolongation of life, but rather with whether that life is, indeed, healthier . . . At the very least, the evidence . . . would indicate that there are no grounds for claiming or supposing that the health of the population is indeed improving to the extent that some believe is indicated by overall mortality trends. Indeed there is a strong indication that the situation may be actually deteriorating.[6]

The McKinlays studied statistics for the health of the United States population, comparing its health status at different points in time. This is known as a longitudinal study, and similar work has been carried out on the UK population by Thomas McKeown, Professor of Social Medicine at Birmingham University. These studies provide some indication of the effects of drugs upon our health.

For one type of illness, infectious disease, most people feel quite certain that drugs have saved innumerable lives. The McKinlays comment: 'It is for these diseases that medicine claims most success in lowering mortality.' At the beginning of this century infectious diseases were the main killers; pneumonia, tuberculosis and diphtheria were rightly feared before the advent of antibiotics. But is it really because we have antibiotics that we are so unlikely to die from them today?

In the United States ten major infectious diseases accounted for about a third of deaths at the turn of the century. The decline in these diseases accounts for nearly 40 per cent of the total decline in mortality since 1900. For each of these diseases, tuberculosis, scarlet fever, influenza, pneumonia, diphtheria, whooping cough, measles, smallpox, typhoid and poliomyelitis, it is generally believed that drug treatment of some type has led to a significant reduction in the death rate. But a close examination of the deaths from each of these diseases shows that the death rate was declining *before* relevant drugs were developed. And further that there was no obvious change in the rate of decline when the drugs became available. In fact the only case for which any medical measure appears to have produced a noticable change in the trend is that of poliomyelitis. Although the disease was already declining and death rates were low, development

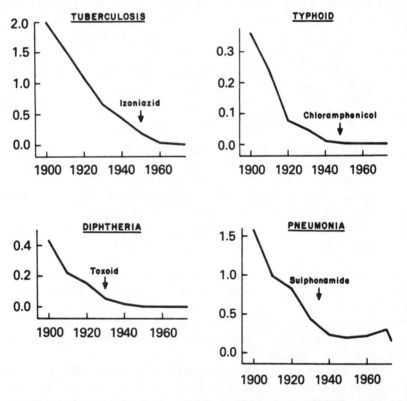

Diagram 7. Fall in the standardised death rate per 1,000 population in relation to specific medical measures. United States 1900–1970. After John and Sonja McKinlay, Ref. 7.

of the Salk vacine in 1955 was accompanied by a fall in the death rate to negligible levels, since when it has virtually disappeared.

Tuberculosis and pneumonia were the two biggest killers of the ten in 1900, and the drugs used for them were part of the antibiotic foundation of the pharmaceutical explosion. Streptomycin and isoniazid, both of which became available in 1950, are still used to treat tuberculosis, but as the graph opposite shows, there was no new fall in death-rate after their introduction.

Sulphonamide, developed in 1935, was used against pneumonia, as were the antibiotics penicillin, tetracycline and the others which followed. Yet between 1950 and 1970 deaths rose slightly, and pneumonia is still an important cause of death in the United States.[7]

The pattern in the United States is mirrored by similar changes in Britain, as McKeown's detailed pioneering work[8] has shown. Looking at trends in death rates from the major infectious diseases during the twentieth century, McKeown found no evidence for any lasting contribution made by medical intervention except in the case of poliomyelitis vaccination, but as in America, polio deaths were already rare when it was introduced. Infectious diseases were in retreat before appropriate drugs were developed.

Tuberculosis mortality in England and Wales shows a trend very similar to that for the United States. The best McKeown could say for medical intervention was that antibacterial drugs reduced the number of deaths by 3.2 per cent over the period since 'cause of death' was first recorded. Vaccination has now been inflicted on generations of reluctant school-children, but tuberculosis was declining before the BCG vaccine was used, and in the Netherlands, where BCG has never been generally accepted, tuberculosis rates fell faster than in Britain.

The introduction of antibiotics made no apparent contribution to the fall in the death rate from pneumonia, bronchitis and influenza, which cannot be separated in British statistics before 1930, although there has been a substantial decline since 1900. The more recent picture for people over the age of sixty-five is grim. McKeown has shown that deaths from pneumonia among the elderly have been rising fast from precisely the time that antibiotics became generally available. The disease has become *more* likely to be lethal to the elderly.

Obviously antibiotics cannot cause pneumonia, but they may indirectly cause death from it. This is simply because we are encouraged to imagine that they offer adequate treatment. Through complacency we may be condemning older people to die from pneumonia in increasing numbers. A second possibile explanation is that we have more vulnerable elderly people. A higher proportion may be bedridden and therefore particularly susceptible to pneumonia. In addition to this, is it possible that the extensive reliance on drug therapy is making old people more feeble? Later in this chapter we shall describe evidence which suggests that this is exactly what is happening.

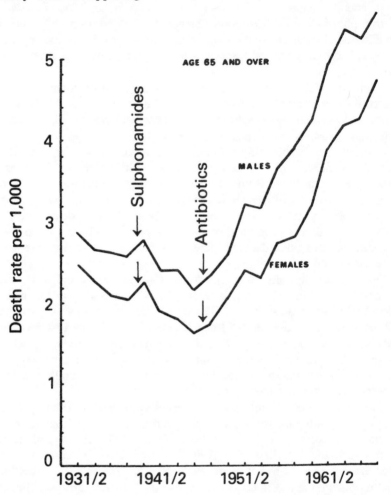

Diagram 8. Pneumonia: mean annual death-rates for England and Wales. After McKeown, Ref. 8.

As we saw in the previous chapter, vast efforts have recently gone into the development of drugs to treat diseases of the cardiovascular system. These have now taken over as the major killers in the developed world, and longitudinal studies of these diseases should provide interesting comparisons with the picture found by McKeown and the McKinlays for the infectious disease.

A World Health Organisation study of trends in deaths due to hyper-tensive disease[9] was unable to find conclusive evidence of benefits of drug therapy. In most countries hypertensive mortality has declined since 1950 when the first drugs to reduce blood pressure were introduced. However, it was at this time that the classification of hypertensive disease as a cause of death came into general use, so clear-cut comparisons between the rate of decline before and after the introduction of the drugs cannot be made. Whilst the improvement in mortality is consistent with the view that it is attributable to these drugs, there is some evidence from Memphis, Tennessee, and from Britain that the decline antedates the drug therapy. It has been suggested that the fall in death-rate from hypertensive disease should be attributed to a reduction in some infectious causes of kidney disease.

International comparisons in changes in hypertensive mortality raise more questions. Whilst most Western countries have experienced a steady decline, in France, Hungary and Yugoslavia mortality has risen dramatic-ally despite the availability of exactly the same drugs. Could it be that the most important influence is lifestyle, and that drugs are largely irrelevant? The evidence cannot be said to be conclusive, but it is highly possible that hypertensive disease, like infectious disease, is not much influenced by the availability of specific forms of drug treatment.

On a wider scale international studies of mortality should show some positive effects of drug use if real benefits exist. Thus comparisons between countries in the developed world where similar drugs are used under similar conditions for identical diseases should show a large degree of uniformity in causes of death. Yet there are significant differences, and the author of the WHO report referred to above comments: 'It is necessary to explain why the mortality trends in countries with apparently similar standards of medical care and availability of drugs should differ to such an extent.' No explanation was offered, but the variation in death rates seems to be attributable to a variety of causes, the effect of which should be comparatively insignificant if drugs were effective.

The medical systems of the United States and Finland are at least as sophisticated as those of Greece, France and Sweden, yet life expectancy for Finnish and American males is much lower. The difference in male death rates from coronary heart disease is startling when Finland is compared with France; in Finland it is five per 1,000 deaths, while in France it is just one per 1,000.[10] Both countries have much the same access to medical knowledge, facilities, drugs and doctors. Why the vastly different heart disease death rate?

Eventually we must all die of something. While the Dutch and the Swiss have the highest cancer rates, Spain and Portugal lead in cerebro-vascular disease (strokes). Sweden and Malta lead in hypertensive heart disease, while the English, Welsh and Romanians expire from a preponderance of respiratory diseases.[11] The reasons for the wide variations in susceptibility to different causes of death are unknown. But such comparisons show quite clearly that the predominant factors at work are geographical, cultural and social. They are of much greater importance than medical intervention.

Another way of trying to identify any benefit from prescribed drugs is to compare prescribing trends with trends in illness. Logically, if prescribing for a particular illness were to increase, eventually that illness should decline, and then prescribing for it would follow its decline. As we have noted, trends in illness are difficult to determine, except when changes are reflected in death rates. However figures for hospitalisation rates can give a reasonable guide.

In the world as a whole, prescribing rates have risen enormously. In Britain specifically, when the NHS was founded, it was believed that the reservoir of untreated sickness would be emptied, and that the population would grow steadily healthier. And this would presumably lead to a steady decrease in the demand for drug therapy. In reality exactly the opposite has been the case.

One common argument in favour of the ready availability of a wide range of prescription drugs is that doctors can treat patients with them in the community instead of sending them to hospital. If this were effective, hospitalisation rates could be expected to have decreased. This does not seem to be the case. In Britain[12] and in the United States[13] days in hospital have risen since the beginning of the pharmaceutical explosion. In both countries, the length of each spell in hospital has decreased, so the increased number of days reflects more separate episodes of illness.

For England and Wales, the rate of hospitalisation in 1958 was seventy-eight per 1,000. Ten years later it had risen to ninety-seven per 1,000, and by 1974 it had reached 103 per 1,000.[14] Possibly patients go into hospital for more minor problems than previously; but surely if drug therapy were highly effective, hospitalisation should now be less necessary for such ailments.

A third type of pointer to any benefits due to prescribed medicines can be found in international comparisons of health facilities. Once more there is a lack of specific knowledge, as international comparisons of drug use are not at present possible because prescribing data are not generally available for most countries. It is a fair assumption, however, that in countries which have more doctors per head of population, and which spend as a consequence more on health, the most sophisticated forms of drug therapy are likely to be readily available to a large proportion of the population.

The eminent epidemiologist Professor Archie Cochrane has investigated questions of this nature, and has produced what has become known as the 'doctor anomaly'. He related age-specific death rates to health facilities in eighteen developed countries, and summarised the findings thus: 'The indices of health care are not negatively associated with mortality.'[15] In other words, more care does *not* mean better health.

If the prevalence of doctors in a particular country is associated with the probability of drug use, Cochrane's findings are nothing less than a horrifying indictment of their principal treatment, chemotherapy. For he showed that 'prevalence of doctors was positively associated with mortality in all age groups except forty-five to fifty-five years, and the association was particularly marked for infant mortality'. And in the latter context supporting evidence that the 'doctor anomaly' in Cochrane's analysis is not an anomaly at all comes from data on perinatal and maternal mortality rates by type of hospital in the United States.[16]

The data comes from the National Study of Maternity Care, a survey by the Committee on Maternal Health of the American College of Obstetricians and Gynaecologists. It shows consistent differences between stillborn, neo-natal death, perinatal and maternal death rates. These differences depend entirely upon the type of hospital involved. Non-teaching hospitals had the lowest death rates on all parameters, followed by non-affiliated teaching hospitals, and then affiliated teaching, with the highest mortality in the medical schools.

The pattern was identical for each variable, with differences ranging from about 30 per cent excess death rate in medical schools for neo-natal death rates, the smallest difference, to a staggering 200 per cent difference in maternal death rates. Non-teaching hospitals show a maternal death rate of 26.3 per 100,000, compared with the medical schools with 52.1 deaths per 100,000. Doris Haire, a formidable American patient advocate, argues from her experience as a special student at the University of Vermont Medical School that these unnecessary deaths occur because 'much of what is done to obstetric patients in hospitals affiliated with medical schools is carried out because a student needs to do it'.[17]

Figures for perinatal mortality in Britain suggest a similar pattern. Marjorie Tew analysed[18] differences between death rates in consultant hospitals, including teaching and other major hospitals, General Practitioner Maternity Units and home births. After meticulous calculations designed to answer the argument that consultant hospitals deal with more difficult and dangerous births, she found that they still showed marked excess in mortality when compared with low-technology deliveries. In Britain today, home births are discouraged; yet Tew's figures show that it is safer to have a baby at home with a minimum of medical intervention than in a consultant hospital.

Doctors, in other words, can be a serious health hazard. And the availability of hospital beds overall has little effect on death rates, which further suggests that the activities of *doctors outside hospitals* are particularly dangerous. The conclusion is inescapable – medication as currently practised is bad for you.

However we assess the evidence the assumed benefits of drug therapy are rarely visible. Antibiotics have saved lives, though fewer than is generally imagined. The beneficial effects of massive medication are dubious when we consider whole populations.

Death rates have been falling in the developed world since the turn of the century and there has been no dramatic drop in recent years in response to increased prescribing. For the USA the graph below shows death rates compared with health expenditure. And the McKinlays argue convincingly[19] that our marginally increased life expectancy is more than counterbalanced by more years of serious disablement. In fact we are not so much living longer, as simply taking a lot longer to die.

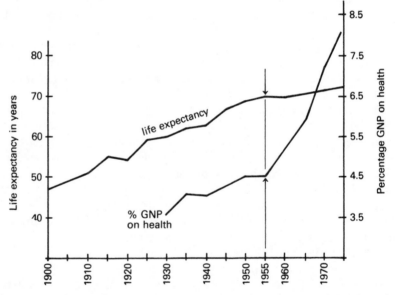

Diagram 9. Life expectancy and health expenditure United States 1900–1973. After John and Sonja McKinlay, Ref. 7.

The McKinlays reached this conclusion by looking at the prevalence of days on which individuals were unable to perform their major daily activity, whether it was work, school, retirement activity or housework, because of illness. By comparing 1964 with 1974 they found that there has been a clear increase in the proportion of the population whose activity was limited. They estimated that the number of restricted activity days per person per year has increased by five for people over forty-five.

In 1964 a man reaching the age of forty-five could expect to live 19.9 more years free of disability. He could then expect a further 7.2 years of life with some disability. A decade later such a man could expect a slight reduction in years free from disability to 19.8, and he could then expect to spend his last 7.9 years disabled. In previous decades the increase in life expectancy for men aged forty-five may have been measurable as a real increase in useful life. Now it has been reduced to a gain in time under disability only. For a woman of forty-five total life expectancy increased by 1.4 years between 1964 and 1974, but life free from disability actually *decreased* by 0.4 years.

This trend can be found for all age and sex groups investigated by the McKinlays except those over sixty-five years, who appear to have experienced small gains in life expected to be free of disability. These estimates of life expectancy without disability are optimistic, because they only allow for limitations in major activity and ignore restrictions caused by illness outside this sphere. For instance, they classify an elderly man capable of keeping himself on his pension outside a nursing home as *not* disabled, even if he were half crippled with arthritis. In view of this, it becomes more clear that recent gains in life expectancy have in practical terms been illusory.

It can be argued that the existence of sickness and disability payments in the developed nations has led to a false increase in the disabled population. After correcting for this possibility the McKinlays found that there was still an unexplained rise in the number of days of restricted activity. They were forced to conclude that between 1964 and 1974 there had been a real increase in the ill health of the population of the United States of America.

In Britain, the government's statistical office carries out yearly surveys of many aspects of everyday life. The information is published as the *General Household Survey* (GHS) and its findings are based on careful representative sampling of the whole British population. Questions about health are normally included in the GHS, but the first detailed study was done in 1977, and there are no comparable data for earlier years. The 1977 GHS however reveals a highly disturbing state of affairs.

With thirty years of free universal health care behind it, Britain should be brimming with vital people whose radiant and wholesome energy is poised to knock the Swedes and the sporting Australians from their mythical positions. At the very least one might expect to find a quietly phlegmatic people, with a firm and unshakable foundation of inner cleanliness, going about their business with a confident sense of their own well-being.

This is not so. Fifty-six per cent of all men and 70 per cent of women reported that they suffered from chronic health problems. Of these, moreover, 67 per cent of the men and 71 per cent of the women reported that they had to take some form of special care *all the time* because of their chronic ill health. In rough round figures, this means that of a population of 56 million, 35 million people now consider themselves chronically ill. And 24 million of the population of Britain are constantly preoccupied with the special care they need because of their poor health.

Within this special care category of weakened and enfeebled individuals are the 33 per cent of men and 40 per cent of women who constantly have to use some form of medication for their chronic health problems: a grim picture of a continually moving river of medication and a mountain of pills that does not include prescriptions for contraceptives. In the great majority of cases these drugs had been prescribed, either by a general practitioner or by a hospital consultant. Relating these figures to the sample as a whole, 18 per cent of all men and 28 per cent of all women are constantly taking prescribed medication – about 15 million people in Britain.

In addition to chronic health problems, the GHS covered short-term health problems. It was found that over half the sample reported some short-term condition which they considered to be independent of any chronic problem. As with chronic ill health, the most common action taken by those with short-term afflictions was to take medication: 45 per cent of men and 49 per cent of women had done so within the previous two weeks. Although most of this was non-prescribed, over-the-counter medicine, about 9 per cent of the short-term sick had consulted their GPs within this period.

It must be the saddest condemnation of Britain's National Health Service that only 23 per cent of men and 15 per cent of women were able to report that there was nothing wrong with them at all. They recalled neither chronic health problems, nor any other sort of ill health in the fourteen days prior to the interview. One is left perversely wondering why – why are *they* healthy? However the information is viewed, the conclusion remains that there has been a major failure when less than one quarter of the population see themselves as healthy. If some cosmic farmer were reviewing his stock in Britain he might conclude that the only sensible course would be to put the lot down and start again.

In Australia, reports on the extent of morbidity in the home environment are sobering. Dr Bridges-Webb found in a random sample survey of families in a Victoria county town that only 11 per cent of those interviewed had no injury, illness or disability to report, or had not taken some medication during the preceeding two weeks. In another context a sample survey of one in eighty households in the metropolitan area of Brisbane revealed that 15 per cent of the respondents, with a predominance of women over men, suffered some disability due to chronic illness. And 8 per cent of all respondents, 18 per cent within the chronic disability group, admitted to suffering from 'nervous or personality disorders'.[20]

The benefits of modern medical practice may be elusive, but their costs are not. Britain spends £144 each year on the NHS for every man, woman and child. Of this total £18 is spent on drugs, filling the average six prescriptions annually used by each individual. But by international standards the country spends relatively little per head of population on health, less than the United States, West Germany or Sweden, for example.[21] A US National Health Care Expenditure Study reported that 60.7 per cent of the American population had prescriptions filled in 1977. The average number of prescriptions per person was 7.2, ranging from 3.5 for the six- to eighteen-year-old group to 14 for people over sixty-five.[22] The pharmaceutical industry expects $8,300 million to have been spent on prescription drugs at retail pharmacies in 1981.[23]

Everywhere health agencies have been committed to primary care policy that involves the almost exclusive use of prescription drugs. Whilst the illnesses we now suffer have a multiplicity of causes, involving social, psychological and physiological factors modified by our cultural and physical environments, there is little doubt that our primary care also creates substantial ill health.

It is difficult to put precise figures on the prevalence of drug-induced disease. There are some indications that specific iatrogenesis is directly related to the rising consumption of drugs, although none of the available evidence is adequate to confirm this in isolation. But when all the evidence is put together, a coherent picture begins to emerge.

We have discussed the promotion of antihypertensive drugs in some detail in an earlier chapter. There has been a massive upsurge in prescribing of these products in Britain which gathered momentum at the beginning of the 1970s, and continued through the decade. British hospital statistics give some indication of one of the possible results. Antihypertensive medication is characterised by adverse effects on the metabolism of the body. Diuretics, often the first mode of attack, can cause metabolic disease, particularly problems associated with mineral depletion. These drugs are also given more to men than to women. And men are now experiencing a great upsurge in metabolic disease: an increase of 50 per cent over sixteen years.

In 1958 there was 22,000 hospital spells due to such ailments, in 1968 the figure had risen to 30,000, and by 1974 it had reached 36,000.[24] Is there a direct connection?

Disease of the blood and blood-forming organs have a well-documented history of medical induction. One of the earliest studied drug hazards was the fatal aplastic anaemia caused by the antibiotic chloramphenicol. Other forms of blood disorder may be caused by a great range of more casually used drugs. As one might expect, some types are all too comon. Anti-inflammatories, antihistamines, antidiabetics, phenothiazines and diuretics have all been implicated as causative agents. Aldomet (methyldopa), the antihypertensive so well advertised and promoted to treat asymptomatic hypertension ('Just two extra minutes of your time could add years to his life . . .') will cause one person in two hundred taking it to develop overt haemolytic anaemia, which can occasionally be fatal. The breakdown of the red blood cells may be severe enough to require blood transfusions and the use of corticosteroids.[25] Corticosteroids in turn are now the principal cause[26] of Cushing's Syndrome, a once rare disease recognisable in the 'moon faces' of its victims. They suffer from water retention, bone fragility, total inability to deal with any shock, and a broad spectrum of other serious symptoms.

Hospitalisation rates for disease of the blood rose by nearly 50 per cent between 1958 and 1968, although they have levelled off at the higher rate since.[27]

Hospital admissions give a more tangible indication of the prevalence of drug-induced disease. A decade ago Commissioner Ley of the FDA stated that 1,500,000 United States hospital admissions annually are attributable to adverse reactions to drugs. Once in hospital, one patient in three is affected by adverse drug reactions.[28]

Studies of the incidence of adverse reactions give widely varying estimates of their prevalence. Some of the variability results from the differences in the methods used; those studies that depend on retrospective reviews of patients' notes not surprisingly show low rates, whilst much higher rates – and more reliable data – have been reported where all patients entering a hospital are carefully monitored.

This method is used in the most extensive and influential of projects investigating drug reactions in hospital, the Boston Collaborative Drug Surveillance Program. It is coordinated by Dr Herschel Jick and his colleagues, and it began as a study of five Boston (Massachusetts) hospitals. The project grew to include six US hospitals and eleven in other countries and it has provided detailed information on a full range of drugs. Nurses record drug use and medical events during each patient's stay in hospital and the information is collated in Boston.[29]

Dr Jick reported that about 31 per cent of all hospitalised patients on the medical wards suffered adverse effects that were probably or definitely drug related. In 80 per cent of the cases, the reaction was rated as moderate or severe.[30]

There is a clear relationship between the number of drugs administered and adverse reaction rates; 4.2 per cent of patients receiving fewer than five drugs, but 45 per cent of patients taking twenty-one or more drugs, were found in one study to suffer adverse reactions.[31] British patients may run a lower risk than their American counterparts; an intensive monitoring study[32] in a group of Scottish hospitals found that each patient receives an average of 4.3 drugs, while it has been estimated that United States hospital patients are given eight or more different drugs.[33] Iatrogenesis rates discovered in different hospitals will reflect variation due to different medication policies.

Drug reactions can significantly prolong hospitalisation. A patient suffering an adverse reaction is likely to stay in hospital about twice as long as a comparable patient with the same disease but no adverse reaction. Consqeuently, in the United States, one-seventh of hospital days are devoted to the care of drug toxicity[34] at a financial cost of many billions of dollars a year and an incalculable cost in human suffering.

A particularly disquieting report from the Boston Collaborative Drug Surveillance Program indicated that the rate of fatal reactions in hospital medical patients was 0.44 per cent.[35] If this figure is extrapolated to the whole of the United States, it implies an annual total of over 130,000 deaths due to drugs among hospital patients.[36] Not all these deaths are avoidable; death due to medication occurs most often among patients who were seriously, possibly fatally, ill. Drug toxicity may be the final straw for elderly patients who would not, in any case, have survived much longer. But the seriousness of the situation must not be dismissed. An editorial in the *New England Journal of Medicine* lamented: 'All of us have seen too much serious illness from drugs for which the patient had no real need.'[37]

Outside hospital wards where it is impossible for nurses to monitor patients constantly, iatrogenesis is more difficult to assess. Many minor drug reactions and sometimes even serious illness are not brought to the doctor's attention. Instead patients may try to ignore their new symptoms or treat them with over-the-counter medicines. If they suspect a drug to be the cause of their symptoms they may simply give up taking the medicine without mentioning it.

When doctors are particularly alert to the risk of adverse reactions they often still fail to detect them. In a study of adverse reactions to cytotoxic drugs, the interviewers (nurses and a cancer specialist) detected toxic effects in eighteen of twenty patients while clinicians recognised them in only twelve. The authors comment in their report that 'non-disclosure of toxicity misleads clinicians about the consequences of treatment'.[38]

Those adverse reactions which are brought to a doctor's notice are all too frequently dismissed as trivial or their iatrogenic basis is denied. The underlying reasons for this situation are discussed later in this book. For the present, it is sufficient to note that iatrogenesis is not among the principal concerns of most physicians. One British doctor who has investigated the level of iatrogenesis in his Peak District practice is Cedric Martys, who has published the results of his two-year detailed study of patients taking any drug for the first time.[39]

Dr Martys included only those patients who were on single drug treatment for relatively straightforward conditions; most were not seriously ill. Each patient was seen after one week's experience with the drug and asked about possible drug side-effects. As the survey specifically excluded multiple drug use and was designed to detect only adverse reactions with short latency – that is, those which showed in a very short time – it is likely to produce a gross underestimate of the problem among this doctor's patients.

Nevertheless, 41 per cent of the patients studied suffered a reaction which was 'certainly' or 'probably' due to the drug prescribed. Adverse reactions were most common with drugs acting on the central nervous system (51 per cent), and with antihistamines (45 per cent). Drugs acting on the heart or respiratory system came next (40 per cent), followed by antibiotics (35 per cent), drugs acting on the gut (31 per cent), with nutritional, hormonal, metabolic and 'miscellaneous' bringing up the rear (22 per cent).

These figures show an incidence of adverse reactions which is much higher than any previous reports have suggested. They indicate a heavy burden of drug-induced illness in the community, a burden which must inevitably grow with each increase in prescribing.

Once more there is a data gap. We have not found similar studies for other countries, and it may be that Britain, which suffered the effects of thalidomide and a long and public battle over compensation, is particularly aware of the problem. But in Canada the Quebec Department of Social Affairs has launched a campaign to reduce the province's estimated $100 million expenditure on the treatment of adverse drug reactions.[40] In the United States Sidney Wolfe has calculated that the misuse of antibiotics in hospitals alone produces 55,000 life-threatening adverse reactions each year, from which there are actually 30,000 deaths in patients whose condition was otherwise non-terminal.[41] The evidence that is available may only be the tip of a very lethal iceberg.

Prescribing patterns in developed nations themselves reveal widespread drug-induced disease. Just as the increasing use of antihypertensive drugs is mirrored by rising rates of metabolic disease, so the increased prescribing of drug treatment for drug-induced conditions reflects a growing amount of iatrogenic disease.

One drug that has been picked out for comment[42] by people researching in this area, because of its rapidly rising use in Britain, is orphenadrine hydrochloride (Disipal). It is used to treat drug-induced Parkinson's disease, a problem which is particularly severe among people who take major tranquillizers such as chlorpromazine (Largactil or Thorazine). The

authoritative *British National Formulary* specifically explains that
'Orphenadrine may also have a mood elevating action which can be useful
in the management of phenothiazine-induced Parkinsonism'.[43] Prescriptions for tranquillizing drugs rose by 76 per cent between 1966 and 1975,
and the rise in the prescribing of preparations for Parkinsonism over the
same period was 114 per cent.[44]

Antihypertensive therapy produces another problem which remains
largely hidden. Had our worker in the Aldomet advert ('I've had a bit of
an accident, Doctor . . .') realised that one of the commonest effects of
those blood pressure pills was impotence, he would have probably stormed
out of the surgery. Almost half (43 per cent) of treated male hypertensives
are impotent. It is true that hypertension itself is associated with some
degree of impotence, and this is to be expected since both problems are
caused by stress. But whereas 43 per cent of treated hypertensives are
impotent, the figure for the untreated is only 17 per cent compared with 7
per cent of the normal population of the same age.[45]

There are other problems in the same physiological area. The sperm
count of American men is dropping, and this appears to be closely linked
to exposure to toxic chemicals, including drugs.

The testes are so sensitive to toxins, including pesticides, herbicides and
radioactive isotopes, that it has been seriously suggested, by Dr Channing
Meyer, Chief of Hazards Boards of the National Institute of Occupational
Safety, that sperm count monitoring could be used as a very effective way
to measure the safety of new chemicals or compounds.[46]

While doctors in Western societies have tended to shy away from
sexual problems, adverse drug reactions in other areas are reported to
the appropriate monitoring bodies. Records of these reactions are
compiled by the FDA in America, the Committee on Safety of Medicines
in Britain, the Australian Drug Evaluation Committee, the Adverse
Reaction Monitoring Centre in the Netherlands, the Israeli National
Centre for Drug Monitoring and numerous other similar bodies through
the world.

For various reasons which we shall look at in the next chapter, the
official figures give a very poor idea of the reality of adverse reactions.
When he was Principal Medical Officer of the Committee on Safety of
Medicines (CSM) in Britain, Dr Inman estimated that perhaps only one
per cent of adverse reactions are reported. And the American figure of
110,000 adverse reactions in eleven years[47] is greatly at variance with the
calculation of Dr Sidney Wolfe given earlier for antibiotics alone.

The reported figures do illustrate a trend. In 1975 the CSM received
5,052 reports of adverse drug reactions. For 1976 the figure was 6,490, by
1977 it had reached 11,255 and it had risen to 11,873 in 1978.[48] If Dr
Inman is right about the correction required, this means British patients

are suffering *over one million* adverse reactions each year from a population of 56 million.

At worst an adverse drug reaction can lead to death. It is often difficult for a physician to identify a death as due to the effects of prescribed drugs. Apart from the practical problems, there is also an understandable reluctance to report a therapeutic failure, especially when it is quite acceptable to write 'heart attack' on a death certificate – or 'liver failure'. The possibility that the heart attack was precipitated by tricyclic antidepressants, or the liver failure associated with chlorpromazine, may be easily overlooked. But deaths from ADRs are occasionally reported to the CSM in Britain.

These figures are not released to the public, but a few trusted researchers are allowed access to them. R.H. Girdwood, Professor of Therapeutics in Edinburgh, has reported on these statistics for a seven-and-a-half year period up to October 1971.[49] He comments: 'Obviously, the figures given are at best a rough guide to some possible dangers . . . Undoubtedly, only a fraction of the adverse reactions are reported . . . Inman showed that only six reports of deaths of asthmatics were reported as possibly being to overuse of pressurised aerosol bronchodilators in 1965 and 1966, whereas it has been estimated that over 1,700 deaths may have been attributable to such preparations.' This example suggests that a corrective factor of 283 could be appropriate.

Girdwood found that only eleven drugs had been credited with more than fifty deaths each. Oral contraceptives head the list with 332 deaths, followed by phenylbutazone, used for rheumatism and arthritis, with 217. Then came chlorpromazine, with 102. The list continues with steroids, isoprenaline, phenacetin, aspirin, oxyphenylbutazone, indomethacin, halothane and amitriptyline. Anti-inflammatory analgesics, with 592 deaths, were the group with the highest mortality.

Whilst totals may be spectacular, figures for deaths make more sense if they are related to the number of prescriptions written for the type of drug. The ratio of deaths per million scripts per annum gives a different list, this time headed by relatively rare drugs, such as sodium aurothiomalate, a gold preparation used for rheumatoid arthritis. Of the commonly prescribed drugs, chlorpromazine remains important, with 8.6 deaths per million scripts, as do phenylbutazone and related anti-inflammatories. The beta-blocker propranolol appears with 7.4 deaths; tricyclic antidepressants follow with 3.6 and 2.3 deaths for imipramine and amitriptyline respectively. And methyldopa appears with 1.3 deaths.

Three of the most dangerous categories of drugs are not used for life-threatening diseases. Together the oral contraceptives, the anti-inflammatory analgesics and the psychotropic drugs accounted for 200 reported deaths per year over the period studied by Girdwood. It is acknowledged that these figures represent a massive underestimate, but by how much? Must we multiply the number of deaths by 283 to get a correct figure? With our present system of data gathering and records there is no way of knowing.

Girdwood mentioned the asthma-aerosol tragedy in his introductory paragraphs. He showed that reporting rates were just under one in 300 in two years. Over the full period of the disaster, and after much publicity, eighty-nine deaths were reported against an actual number of 3,500.[50] In this case about forty times as many people died as were reported. If this correction is applied to 'our figure of 200 for the three groups of drugs specified above, then the death toll becomes 8,000 per annum. By 1975, prescribing of these drugs had increased by nearly 50 per cent compared to the period studied by Girdwood. So it could reasonably be that deaths from these drugs alone reached 12,000 each year in Britain by the second half of the 1970s.

What then of the effect of drugs which are acknowledged to be hazardous, and are prescribed for life-threatening conditions? What is the true death rate from these drugs? What is the real effect of massive prescribing of antihypertensives, of beta-blockers and of the increasing trend towards life-long regimes of medication, when the risks build up year after year and the odds progressively shorten?

Even if we could satisfactorily answer these urgent questions they would not give us the whole picture. Drugs cause deaths in more subtle ways. One which would rarely be reported as a drug death is that resulting from the effect of the ubiquitous benzodiazepines (Valium, Librium, Mogadon, Dalmane and so on), on driving ability.

People who take this type of drug have been shown to be at greater than normal risk of road accidents. One study[51] of the drugs taken by fifty-seven people killed while driving showed that they were much more likely to have taken tranquillizers than a matched control group of drivers. The risk of serious road accident is increased by a factor of five. Similarly benzodiazepine sleeping pills cause poor reactions and impaired coordination the morning after they are taken. Driving ability is hindered much more by drug-assisted sleep than by insomnia. And the harmful drug effects are cumulative, mounting up over successive nights.[52]

We are now venturing into the limitless, and highly speculative, area of the social cost of medication. We will only pursue the question a short way. The problems with tranquillizers are becoming known,[53] but what are the real consequences of widespread impotence? There must certainly be costs in terms of marital and relationship breakdown which will have a knock-on effect. Marital problems are the largest cause of suicide, and major contributory factor in delinquency. It is possible that increased use of tranquillizers is also actively contributing to the rising violence of the affluent countires? They have been shown to lead to violent outbreaks, in much the same way as alcohol. Tranquillizers do not make problems go away; they just suppress, up to a point, our reactions to them.

Finally evidence is beginning to emerge that drugs taken by pregnant women,[54] and those administered during labour and delivery of babies, have harmful effects on the mind and behaviour of the offspring:[55] an effect which is horrific, subtle, unseen and – once the drugs are taken – unavoidable. Throughout the Western world social commentators search for the reasons for social breakdown and aberration. Is there a biochemical foundation to this malaise?

We have shown that there is very little evidence that prescribed drugs have led to any increase in life expectancy. Their most highly acclaimed successes have been with the infectious diseases, especially pneumonia, tuberculosis and poliomyelitis. But these diseases were already all in retreat.

Every developed nation has a growing number of older people among its population proportionate to the whole. These survivors reflect the substantial improvements in elementary childcare and the decline of the infectious diseases that occurred over the first half of this century. Crude mortality figures show that more of those born since the First World War will live to old age. But the increased numbers of senior citizens does not reflect a longer average life-span. The biblical three score years and ten is still the rule today.

The decline in death rate during the twentieth century must be attributed predominantly to social, economic and environmental causes, not to drug therapy. International studies have shown that among countries with over \$600 (1965) per head average income, more sophisticated Western medicine leads to higher death rates.[56]

In developed societies such as Britain, thirty years of enormous use of free drug therapy has produced a population in which 70 per cent reports itself suffering chronic ill health. Hospitalisation rates in both the United States and the UK are rising. In the United States, middle-aged people can expect more years of disability and fewer years of active life than they could a decade ago.

The direct effects of drug damage are apparent in the statistics for iatrogenic disease. With the rare exceptions of small intensive surveys, adverse reactions to drugs are enormously underestimated. The best estimates of drug-induced disease in the population of Britain lead to a constant prevalence of 2 per cent, or over one million people.

Drug-induced deaths must be estimated. The probable figure for Britain is between 10,000 and 15,000 deaths in an unexceptional year at the current rate of prescribing. To put this into perspective, road accidents killed 6,790 people in 1978. And in America the hope has been expressed by FDA personnel that drug deaths and damage may soon be reduced to the level suffered in motor accidents.[57]

It seems that medicine's ancient injunction, *non nocere* – do not harm – has been forgotten, or at least lost with a vengeance, beneath mountains of pills and rivers of potions.

Part Two

Taken on Trust

Chapter Seven

Guardian Angels

Many drug firms make the mistake of believing that their chemists can furnish trustworthy pharmacological opinion. Indeed, some eminent chemists, impatient with careful pharmacologic technique, have ventured to estimate for themselves the clinical possibilities of their own synthetics . . . There is no short cut from chemical laboratory to clinic, except one that passes too close to the morgue.

– A pharmacologist speaking at the 1929 meeting
of the Section of Pharmacology and Therapeutics
of the American Medical Association

Although judgements . . . may reasonably differ, all judgements are made from the same foundation – scientific data. If the integrity of that data is questioned, then the whole regulatory process is questioned. If the data are proven false and misleading then the regulatory decision may be tragically wrong.

– Senator Edward Kennedy at the Joint Hearings
before the Senate Subcommittee on Health,
January 1976

Unacceptable drug disasters compounded by the unethical behaviour of some manufacturers have forced governments to institute controls over the medicines used in their countries. A totally political dimension was created in the production and use of drugs. Governments found themselves having to inhibit the activities of industries they would otherwise wish to encourage, and this has led to unsatisfactory compromise.

In most countries the thalidomide disaster was the watershed. Before it, drug companies were more or less free to manufacture and sell whatever they liked. They would prefer to revert to a situation where they are trusted to do what they consider best with the minimum of bureaucratic control.[1]

Regulation generally covers the following areas: the licensing of new drugs; the assessment of drugs which are already on the market; the control and use of each drug; and the monitoring of drug effects, particularly adverse reactions. Many poor countries rely on second-hand regulation, following the pattern established in developed nations with which they have economic or social ties.

The control systems vary between nations, both in emphasis and in the power given to the regulatory agency. Each nation tends to regard the use of the products of the multinational drug companies as a purely domestic matter. So there is little compatibility between agencies, and a decision reached about a drug in one country will frequently be at variance with that reached in another, even when each considers the same evidence.

The Food and Drug Administration of the United States (the FDA) has both a comparatively long history and considerable independence and authority. Increasingly its actions are being challenged and reversed in the courts, a problem which reflects its unusual willingness to make contentious decisions in the face of strong opposition from the pharmaceutical industry.

The FDA's recent regulatory history began with disaster. Evidence of the safety of new drugs was not required prior to the passage of the Food, Drugs and Cosmetic Act of 1938.[2]

In 1937, the S.E. Massengill Company of Tennessee, pausing only to check the flavour, fragrance and appearance of their product, marketed a new variation of an anti-bacterial sulphanilamide. The drug had been previously available in tablet and capsule forms, but Massengill's sales staff reported demand for a liquid form that children could take more easily. Sulphanilamide would not readily dissolve in any of the usual drug carriers. This problem was overcome by using diethylene glycol, the principal constituent of anti-freeze; and 240 gallons of this elixir were made and marketed.

Shortly afterwards the FDA were informed that eight children with sore throats and one adult with gonorrhoea had died after taking the medicine. When the company heard of the poisonings it sent out over a thousand telegrams in an effort to recall the lethal mixture. Large amounts were recovered, but eventually over two hundred FDA personnel were needed on the ground, and radio and press appeals and warnings were issued.

In spite of the lives at risk and the urgency of the task, some physicians, chemists and salesmen proved obstructive, refusing to breach confidentiality by releasing the names of patients. Over a hundred people died. Autopsies revealed fatal damage to the liver and kidneys.

The American Medical Association (AMA) requested the formula for the mixture, which was supplied by Massengill with a plea for confidentiality. Some days later the company telegraphed the AMA: 'Please wire . . . suggestion for antidote and treatment', to which the AMA could only respond, 'Antidote for Elixir Sulfanilamide-Massengill not known . . .'

The tragedy occurred during the period from June to October 1937. On the 23rd October, Dr Massengill issued this press statement:

My chemists and I deeply regret the fatal results, but there was no error in manufacture of the product. We have been supplying legitimate professional demand and not once could have foreseen the unlooked-for results. I do not feel that there was any responsibility on our part. The chemical sulfanilamide had been approved for use and had been used in large quantities in other forms, and now its bad effects are developing.[3]

This early small-scale disaster contained all the essential elements of similar events today. Product innovation under commercial pressure; inadequate knowledge and testing of clinical effects; ineffective monitoring and recall; a denial of ethical standards of professional behaviour; refutation of responsibility by the manufacturer; and the quiet disposal of the dead – including Massengill's chief chemist, who committed suicide. Little has changed in the following forty years.

Perhaps it would be naive to expect change. Regulation is, by definition, a retrospective process. It would be unrealistic to expect anybody to propose regulations that could cope with every unwanted possibility. Control is aimed at preventing the recurrence of a previously unpredicted disaster. With accumulated experience some rules and procedures emerge that may help to prevent more generalised types of disaster. But with any innovative technology there is bound to be unforseen risk. Jim Morrison of the FDA said, 'Science changes faster than we can write the regulations.'

In the United States, this experience is reflected in the Code of Federal Regulations. Section 21, parts 1 to 1300, state in explicit detail the procedures with which drug manufacturers must comply in a wide variety of circumstances. These range from the procedure for obtaining approval for a new drug to the precise details of envelope size and type face to be used for warning letters to doctors. They are the most comprehensive regulations in the world.

The FDA was part of the United States Government Department of Health, Education and Welfare (HEW), now Department of Health and Human Services. It is concerned with anything we put in or on ourselves – cosmetics, food additives and household products as well as medicines. One section of the FDA, the Bureau of Drugs, deals specifically with pharmaceuticals. Within the Bureau of Drugs is a proliferation of sub-divisions such as the Division of Drug Experience, New Drug Evaluation, the Division of Scientific Investigations, and the Division of Drug Advertising, each with its own Director and team of specialist staff. Advisory committees are recruited from outside the FDA, with members invited on the basis of particular expertise.

The operation of the FDA is meticulous. The mode of action of the Division of Drug Advertising is typical. If it requires the modification of an advertisement to comply with regulations, this may be done on the telephone between people who know each other, but the substance of the conversation will become a matter of public record through the exchange of confirmatory letters. If the low-key approach should fail, the Bureau can resort to enforcement via the courts after establishing the exact nature of the violation.

The Division has the power to demand corrective advertising. On one occasion a company was asked to display two remedial advertisements to counter an acknowledged infringement. After complying with this, the company ran a third advertisement which repeated the original violation. The FDA obtained a seizure order through the court for the products advertised.

Perhaps owing to some misunderstanding when the term 'drugs' was transmitted from the FDA in Washington to New York, things got slightly out of hand. A sheriff, with posse armed with machine guns, captured the warehouse and everyone in it, as well as $1.5 million worth of the company's stock. Under normal circumstances, the work of the Bureau is best characterised as the maintenance of a perpetual watching brief.[4]

Before any drug can be marketed in the United States it must be approved for its intended use by the FDA. This is done through the submission of a New Drug Application (NDA) by the manufacturer or his agent. The New Drug provisions of the Food, Drugs, and Cosmetic Act require that a manufacturer submit evidence demonstrating the *safety* of its products before introducing them into the market. This statute was strengthened by the Kefauver-Harris Amendment of 1962 which added the requirement that substantial evidence of *effectiveness* from clinical investigations must also be submitted for FDA approval.

The FDA itself does very little drug toxicity testing, and no clinical trials. Its task is to define the tests it believes necessary and to determine whether or not new products comply. For each NDA, specific pieces of information are required. These include a full statement of the drug's composition and a description of the methods used in, and the facilities and controls used for, the manufacturing, processing and packing of the drug. Samples of the drug and its components are required, and specimens of the proposed labelling. But the bulk of the NDA comprises reports of investigations designed to show that the new drug is both safe and effective.[5]

Initial testing is carried out on animals and animal tissues. Acute and prolonged toxicity testing will establish the LD 50, the dose of drug that is lethal to 50 per cent of animals of a variety of species, from mice and rabbits to dogs and monkeys. Lengthy and thorough testing for carcinogenic (cancer-causing) properties is demanded, as are tests on pregnant animals to indicate any teratogenic effects. Smaller doses of the drug are used to investigate therapeutic and other effects, and to determine dose-response relationships. Both physiological and behavioural effects are studied, and changes looked for in the test animals' various organs and systems. Behavioural studies are likely to include measures of the animals' activity, from sleep at one extreme to agitation at the other; their sensitivity to stimuli; and their learning ability. From the animal work, the new drug's possible therapeutic value and approximate dose necessary to produce the desired effects are judged.

The FDA is allowed thirty days from receipt of animal data in which to decide either to reject the application or to allow the company to proceed with testing the new drug on people.

Clinical trials, first with volunteers, then with larger and less critical groups of patients, are designed to establish the precise parameters of use for the drug, its therapeutic effects and to show up adverse reactions. If these trials are deemed to have demonstrated that the drug meets the requirements of the law, and the manufacturer's claims, it will be approved and allowed onto the market.

There are problems with this system of drug approval. A fundamental difficulty is that the regulatory agency has to make an assessment of a drug which is based on someone else's report: an assessment of an assessment. And those who provide the original information, the drug manufacturers, are not always as honest or unbiased as might be hoped.

The Senate Subcommittee hearings under Edward Kennedy on Preclinical and Clinical Testing by the Pharmaceutical Industry in 1976[6] left little doubt on this. Questions raised on the data submitted by G.D. Searle & Co. relating to their drugs Flagyl and Aldactone caused the FDA to send teams of inspectors to check Searle data back as far as 1968 on twenty-five selected drugs.

During the hearings, Alexander Schmidt MD, Commissioner of the FDA, commented that, 'The required attention to detail in conducting these animal studies is sometimes lacking.' He considered that this was 'a general problem throughout the industry'. On the Searle data, Commissioner Schmidt reported that the firm 'had presented no less than three volumes of Corrected and Expanded Reports which had been prepared by Searle scientists to identify differences between the initial reports submitted to the FDA and the actual data. He went on: 'It is disconcerting that even today, after three separate reviews by Searle personnel of the same data from the 78-week rat study, we are continuing to discover errors that complicate review of this study.'

In evidence, Dr Schmidt cited examples of test animals developing malignant tumours which were not reporteed, of animals having corrective surgery and remaining in tests, of tissue reports not corresponding with the actual data, of examinations reported which had not been carried out, and 'errors in documentation too numerous to mention'.

The hearings were not without their lighter moments. At one point, Senator Kennedy asked Dr Schmidt: 'If you cannot get a person to tell whether the animal is dead or alive, what kind of value are you going to give to their analysis about whether it is a cancer-causing agent?' Senator Beall remarked 'It's interesting to note that one of these [record sheets on test mice], B14MF, says that it was killed on July 30th, 1971, and alive on October 19, 1971 – apparently it was not an effective hit job.'

The FDA memo on its findings on the Searle data lists six major points of criticism and notes thirty-seven other criticisms concerning Flagyl, Norpace, Cu7 (Copper 7 intra-uterine device, or coil), Ovulen and Enovid. It also records delays of *four to six years* in forwarding information to the FDA.

In summary, Dr Schmidt said:

> I think that we found deficiencies and errors essentially in all of the twenty-five studies . . . Because of the perfunctory nature of the observations, tissue masses come and go and animals die more than once. Necropsy reports submitted to the FDA are frequently at variance with raw data. Unexplained alterations are made by unidentified persons in both antemortem and postmortem records. Apparent lack of firm direction at the corporate level of the pathology-toxicology department and regulatory affairs staff to ensure the credibility of studies and submissions to the FDA.

Inadequate data submission can have serious consequences. In 1962 Richardson-Merrill possessed animal test data on a new cholesterol-lowering drug, code-named Mer-29. Had this been submitted in accurate form, the drug's capacity to cause cataract could have been recognised earlier. However, it was not, and about a thousand people suffered eye damage. The company had criminally suppressed laboratory observations of cataract formation, hair loss and gonadal changes in rats and dogs. Richardson-Merrill was fined $80,000 by the District Court in Washington DC for withholding and falsifying test data.[7]

After animal tests have been accepted the next major hurdle is the clinical trial. There is no substitute for using the drug on man, for no matter how rigorous the animal test procedures, some effects will slip through. Practolol passed all the required animal tests; and with thalidomide it was found that the polyneuritis it induced is unique to man, and some effort was necessary to reproduce its foetus-deforming effect in laboratory animals.[8] This is not because man is especially sensitive or complicated; species-specific drug effects are frequently found. For instance, a minute dose of LSD can cause the body temperature of a rabbit to rise so high that the animal will die, but this effect has not been found in any other animal.[9] Codeine causes convulsions in cats which are often fatal. Such effects could have prevented some drugs from being used in man.

There is an underlying criticism of all clinical trials. It is that the information and results of such trials is routed through the drug manufacturers. This inevitably throws doubt on the validity of any results. If the data produced by one specialist are not quite what was hoped for, it is quite in order for the company to continue trials elsewhere until satisfactory results and testimonials are achieved. Negative results are very rarely published and indeed some clinicians tell of pressure to keep quiet about such data.[10]

A drug manufacturer will arrange appropriate clinical trials by approaching sympathetic medical consultants whose interests lie in areas relevant to the intended application of the drug. The drug will be given to volunteers or patients under the consultant's supervision, and he will report the effects to the company. Naturally he is paid a substantial fee for his work.

On the face of it, this would seem to be a reasonable system. In practice it is not. Some consultants are more conscientious than others, and the whole process is open to subjective interpretation.

Glowing testimonials were obtained for the clinical efficacy and safety of thalidomide; even Dr McBride, who eventually uncovered its effects on the unborn child, gave the drug a recommendation on the basis of the clinical observations he made as an obstetrician at Sydney's prestigious Crown Street Women's Hospital.[11]

Essentially the physician's task is to judge whether the patient's condition is improved after use of the drug. Many subtle pitfalls can hinder arrival at a correct assessment. One is the placebo effect, by which the patient may respond equally well to an inert substance as to a drug. And the physician's knowledge of the drug's expected effect can influence both his patient's state and his judgement of the trial. Many other questions arise. Is the group of experimental patients typical of the patient population that will be treated with the drug? Is the consultant competent to observe drug effects outside his field of specialisation? Has he devised appropriate statistical tests to interpret his results?

Problems with clinical trials are universally acknowledged. Professor Archie Cochrane, who has studied the problem internationally, believes that most northern European countries are on a par. West Germany is an anomaly where the medical profession consider that carrying out a clinical trial is not a suitable occupation for gentlemen, so the drug manufacturers do them. In the Mediterranean countries, medical students receive very little training in scientific method. This could have far-reaching effects if the EEC establishes common criteria for drug acceptance.

Nowhere in the world are clinicians well trained in experimental design, statistical analysis, or other crucial aspects of scientific method. Yet their *opinions* are the key to the marketing of every new drug.

Lack of time for clinical trials limits their value. Drug tests lasting a matter of weeks will not give unambiguous results. Some substances may have fatal effects which take years to emerge, like the cancer caused by asbestos. It is obvious that clinical trials which will give an accurate picture of all the effects of a drug are beyond most medical institutions. Occasionally there will be effects beyond the scope of any clinical trial. The synthetic female hormone stilboestrol (DES) damages the sons and daughters of mothers to whom it was given. No trial would have indicated the way in which this was to happen, although damage to the offspring of rats exposed to pre-natal DES was observed and reported in 1940.[12]

The dishonesty of some of the physicians carrying out trials is a major problem. The FDA's concern about this issue led in 1976 to the establishment of a Bio-research Monitoring Program (Bi-Mo). The need for Bi-Mo became apparent in the early 1960s, when it was observed that 'a small stable of clinical investigators were contributing to a great many new drug applications seemingly outside of their field of competence.'

The first investigator to be investigated was a general practitioner who had undertaken clinical studies for twenty-five companies, covering a wide range of products and applications. The FDA found that this doctor had submitted false, fraudulent and fictitious reports in support of five NDAs. He was the first of some thirty-six in the USA to have been declared ineligible to receive shipments of investigational new drugs.[13]

Michael Hendsley, of the Office of Scientific Investigations at the FDA, has emphasised that it was not just private doctors but prestigious academics who had flouted test protocols, falsified data and submitted phony consent documents.

The FDA is not willing to give the names of these doctors, although if asked whether a particular individual has been found guilty of this sort of behaviour, they will answer. One investigator identified as 'Dr 31', was found to have submitted data to one sponsor company which was identical to that submitted to another company on another drug. When confronted by the FDA inspectors, he explained that he was such a 'compulsive worker' that he had taken the original data with him on a picnic and that they had been lost when his rowing boat capsized. This story was disproved when the FDA learned that 'Dr. 31' had tried to persuade a nurse to say she had been in the boat at the time.[14]

The Bi-Mo Program now has records of some 80,000 clinical investigators which it continually sifts for irresponsible practice. Dr Frances Kelsey, who heads this task force, feels that although its existence has led to improved performance in clinical trials and better patient and volunteer protection, the number of clinical investigators disqualified is a simple function of the number of staff members available to her. The more she investigates, the more clinicians are disqualified.

A totally satisfactory drug trial requires enormous resources and would be impossible for any solo clinician. Such a trial[15] was organised by the World Health Organisation and involved the ICI drug clofibrate, marketed as Atromid-S. Since its introduction in 1963 sales had climbed well and clofibrate was a good export earner. The drug reduces cholesterol levels in the blood and the object of its use is to protect those who take it from vascular disease. To measure the effectiveness of clofibrate, the World Health Organisation set up a multi-national team of specialists working in Edinburgh, Prague and Budapest. Some 15,745 volunteers participated, accumulating a total of 83,534 treatment years' experience with the drug between them. It is a study unequalled in scale and thoroughness.

The main finding to emerge was that those taking the drug had a higher death-rate than those who were not. Also, clofibrate did reduce the incidence of *non-fatal* heart attacks, but it did not affect the incidence of *fatal* attacks. The higher death-rate had many causes, usually apparently unconnected with the treatment but an excess of serious digestive and gall bladder problems stood out among those who had taken clofibrate.

The results were first published in 1978 by an international group of cardiologists. The West German government reacted by immediately banning the drug pending an assessment of its use, and in Norway it was restricted to licensed hospital use only. The governments of these countries had gone further than the cautious authors of the report, who had concluded that 'Clofibrate cannot be recommended as a lipid (cholesterol) lowering drug for community-wide primary prevention of ischaemic heart disease'.

The rigour of this WHO study did not convince ICI that its conclusions were justified. As late as August 1980, when the persistent hazards of clofibrate treatment were confirmed in a follow-up report in the *Lancet*,[16] ICI continued to deny that the higher death-rate was due to the drug.[17] Because its effect is of a previously unknown type – possibly accelerated ageing – some pharmacologists doubt whether the trial results should be applied to clofibrate when used for patients with lipid-related problems.

Whatever the weaknesses, the acceptance of clinical data is generally the final step before a new drug can be marketed. Once a drug is established the permitted indications for its use can be extended through further clinical trials. This is an essential part of the 'spread of indications' strategy employed by the manufacturers to increase the potential market for each product.

All the problems with the integrity of the original trials will continue with subsequent tests. Clinical trials which could clear the way for promotion of an established drug for more patients have enormous financial value. This is illustrated by the case of Geigy's Anturan (sulphinpyrazone), a drug prescribed on a fairly small scale for gout.

Anturan was the subject of a major clinical trial[18] designed to demonstrate its effectiveness in preventing sudden death due to a subsequent heart attack in patients who had suffered myocardial infarction. Obviously, if it could be established that Anturan did reduce mortality in these high-risk patients, it would have unique value. When the results of the multicentre trial were reported to the regulatory bodies in Britain and the United States, they came to different conclusions about their validity. In Britain, the CSM accepted Anturan and it is now prescribed for heart patients. In America, the more cynical FDA rejected the trial and refused permission for Geigy to market the drug as a prophylactic. The FDA's main objections to the Anturan re-infarction trial were summarised in a disturbing Special Report which appeared in the *New England Journal of Medicine* in December 1980.[19]

The FDA gave three broad reasons for its decision. First, the major finding of the trial (reduction in sudden death among patients treated with Anturan) was based on a classification of cardiac deaths into three categories: sudden death, acute myocardial infarction, or other cardiac event. The reviewers discovered that assignments were often inaccurate and that they failed to conform with the criteria set at the outset of the study. The assignment errors nearly all favoured the conclusion that Anturan decreased sudden death. Second, the classification scheme had no clear logic and did not divide deaths into meaningful or discrete groups. Essentially identical case histories could lead to diverse classifications.

Finally, the FDA found that the reported effect on overall mortality depended heavily on *post hoc* exclusion from the analysis of results for patients who had participated fully in the study and died while receiving therapy. When all patients were included, there was only a very weak trend showing slight improvement with Anturan which could have been due to chance.

Once a drug has been approved for marketing, the interest of the regulatory body diminishes. Yet is it not until a drug is in widespread use that many of its unwanted effects will emerge. Regulatory agencies are usually involved in collecting information about drugs in use. This is a fairly recent development even in the United States. It was only after thalidomide that the FDA established a registry for suspected adverse drug reactions; physicians and drug manufacturers are now required by law to report any suspected case to the Bureau of Drugs.

The FDA definition of an adverse drug reaction (ADR) includes 'any adverse experience associated with the use of the drug, whether or not considered drug-related, and any side-effect, injury, toxicity or sensitivity reaction, or significant failure of expected pharmacologic action'. Other bodies rely on the WHO definition, which is both simple and broad: a drug effect 'which is noxious and unintended, and which occurs at doses normally used in man for the prophylaxis, diagnosis or therapy of disease, or for the modification of physiological function.'[20]

However they are defined, adverse reactions are difficult to identify. Dr Judith Jones, Director of the Division of Drug Experience at the FDA, has listed three factors which inhibit detection. These are:

1 Difficulty in differentiating the purported reaction from underlying diseases, or negative placebo effects.
2 The silent nature of many ADRs. If they are not specifically looked for, they will not be found: for example, kidney and liver damage.
3 Difficulty in identifying which drug in typical multi-drug regimes may be reasonably causing the suspected reaction.

One consequence is that only the cruder ADRs get picked up and reported.

The FDA has two standard forms for reporting adverse reactions. These are submitted as confidential documents, and the names of the patient, physician and hospital involved remain confidential. Despite legal sanctions and protection, this is recognised as a low-yield system. It requires high motivation on the part of physicians and exemplary concern on the part of the drug manufacturers to get the forms filled in and back to the FDA. Around 12,000 reports are received each year, and although useful on a nationwide basis to warn of rare and dramatic effects, they do not give reliable data on the incidence of ADRs.[21]

Reports received by the FDA are classified on arrival according to the seriousness of the particular type of reaction, and previous knowledge of it. Any previously unknown or serious ADR is further investigated, its causality and biological plausibility evaluated, and corroborating evidence collated. Occasionally, reports are checked back to their source by field agents. More usually, however, the reports are fed straight into a computer data-handling system which allows access to information under various headings, such as disease, type of drug and type of ADR. From the computerised data the pharmacological profile of each drug is developed, and the broad spectrum of its effects characterised. The computer profile of Merck, Sharp & Dohme's antihypertensive agent, Aldomet (methyldopa) includes one hundred separate adverse effects, divided into ten categories covering almost all body systems.[22]

Periodic reviews of the computer data bank on ADRs leads to action when it is considered appropriate. Case control studies may be initiated; these involve identifying people who suffer from a particular disease and searching for the suspected cause in their drug history. Often this is the only way a delayed adverse reaction can be detected; but it is not likely to reveal a previously unsuspected relationship. In one recent case-control study,[23] women admitted to hospital after heart attacks were asked whether they had ever taken oral contraceptives. It was found that these women were more likely to be Pill users than a comparison group of women hospitalised for other types of illness, and also that heart attack patients who were not current oral contraceptive users were more likely to have taken the Pill *in the past* than control group women.

The first drug to be banned totally by the FDA was phenformin, an oral anti-diabetic agent. On 25th July 1977, Health, Education and Welfare Secretary Joseph Califano announced that phenformin constituted an 'imminent hazard to the public health'. Califano was urged to take this action in a petition from Dr Sidney Wolfe, who heads Ralph Nader's Health Research Group. The petition was filed because of continuing deaths from lactic acidosis, an adverse reaction to phenformin which is fatal to half its victims. Lactic acidosis has been known for twenty years, but powerful members of the medical profession argued that phenformin was a useful drug. Despite criticism of the ban by the American Medical Association, it was upheld by FDA commissioner Donald Kennedy in November 1978 and the manufacturers have not contested the decision.[24]

The FDA drug data base is increasingly used for risk/benefit assessment of drugs in use and for drug epidemiology studies. One refinement in the detection of unwanted drug effects is SOAR – Screening of Adverse Reactions.[25] This programme organises reports of ADRs into nineteen body systems – for example, digestive, nervous, cardiac, etc. – so that adverse drug event patterns can be seen more readily. Then, using data supplied by a research organisation which monitors sales through pharmacies and drug wholesalers, a drug use profile is constructed for each drug. Adverse reactions in a particular body system for each drug are compared with patterns for other, similar drugs in the same class. When the proportion of ADRs relative to the quantity of the drug used reaches twice or more the proportion for similar drugs, SOAR produces a warning signal.

SOAR was tested in 1979 using sales data and ADR information gathered between 1973 and 1976. Five drugs were included in the study: erythromycin estolate (Ilosone), clindamycin (Dalacin C), methyldopa (Aldomet), thioridazine (Melleril), ibuprofen (Brufen), and phenformin (eg Dibotin). For most of these drugs, the adverse reactions signalled by SOAR were known before 1973, but some were signalled by the programme at a point before they had actually been recognised. If SOAR had been operational before 1975 it would have given warning of the serious cardiovascular reactions to ibuprofen which led to a modification in its labelling in 1977. SOAR could have acted as an early warning system, showing up this problem two years earlier. Similarly, the relationship between severe colitis and clindamycin would have been signalled in March 1973, well before it became known.[26]

Should a drug prove to have unacceptable hazards, the FDA will take action to restrict its use. Warning letters may be sent directly to doctors in specially designed envelopes, and the FDA will also use public media should it be considered necessary. All regulatory decisions are published and thus are a matter of public debate.

In Britain drug regulation is a post-thalidomide phenomenon. The Committee on Safety of Drugs was set up in 1964; later it became the Committee on Safety of Medicines (CSM). The tone of its work is clearly indicated by its terms of reference, which were:

1 To give *advice* with respect to safety, quality and efficacy, in relation to human use, of any substance or article (not being an instrument, apparatus or appliance) to which any provision of the medicines Act 1968 is applicable.
2 To promote the collection and investigation of information relating to adverse reactions for the purpose of enabling such advice to be given.

Under the Medicines Act of 1968, the CSM is lumped together with Committees on the Review of Medicines, on Dental and Surgical Materials, Veterinary Products, and the Commission of the British Pharmacopoeia. According to the 1978 Report, the CSM has thirty-two subcommittees and two *ad hoc* consultative groups, but only one joint subcommittee and one working party. These posts are filled by 587 people, mainly professors and doctors.[27] They are backed up by a large staff of full-time civil servants whose names are not published.

One might have anticipated that Britain, with the benefit of a late start, and following the deliberations of the Dunlop Committee, would have a tailor-made body designed to avoid the problems experienced by the FDA. But with a characteristic display of national independence, Britain opted to rely on the amateur tradition typified by well-established experts in various fields serving on part-time committees.

The CSM's terms of reference do not mention the medical need for a new drug. Efficacy merely implies that the drug should be superior to a placebo, not that it need be a useful addition to the pharmacopoeia. Nor is there any special attention to innovations of particular therapeutic value. In these respects, the CSM is less discriminatory than some other regulatory bodies. The FDA, for example, handles new drug applications for new chemical entities and those which are claimed to be of significant therapeutic value more quickly than me-too drugs. In contrast, the CSM treats all applications alike.[28] In Norway the regulatory body considers first whether there is an expressed medical need for each new drug; if there is not, the new drug application is rejected without further processing.[29] The CSM has no such powers.

A new drug must be approved by the CSM before it can be marketed in Britain. The procedure is basically the same as that of the FDA, except that there are no published regulations with which manufacturers and products must comply. It all happens in the huddle of committees. The progress of a new drug from the laboratory through the CSM and onto the market is a journey through highly cohesive layers bound by narrow interest and academic insularity. The move from one layer to the next is small, and when a product makes the jump – say from company laboratory to CSM review – it is likely that it will land in sympathetic hands.

Drug regulatory bodies such as the CSM draw their key members from a highly specialised pool. Limited numbers of people occupy the top status and experience brackets, and few are available to fill the positions. Since each institution, whether commercial, academic or bureaucratic, requires its quota of suitable heads, a career merry-go-round develops. This results in a close interaction between institutions, and the possibility of a consequent blurring of functional properties cannot be overlooked.

One effect of this closeness is illustrated by the experience of Dr Cahal, one-time head of the Committee on Safety of Drugs, when he made an error in assessing tabulated information. Through misreading a title he concluded that a new drug could lead to abnormalities when in fact this had not been shown. He was sharply pulled up by the company concerned[30] – a concise example both of the ease of communication and the relative power relationships of the protagonists.

Dr Cahal, now a Senior Principle Medical Officer in the civil service, well recalls the early days of drug monitoring. In the wake of thalidomide, he and five colleagues with two pharmacists and eighteen assistants were given the task of monitoring all adverse drug reactions in Britain, as well as vetting new drugs. Due thought having been given to the scope and importance of the task, they were equipped with ball-point pens, a shoe box, and a supply of postcards.

Today in Britain, adverse drug reactions are monitored by the 'yellow card' system. Every doctor is asked to report every serious or unusual ADR observed in his practice. To facilitate this, he is supplied with pre-addressed and pre-paid yellow cards, designed to enable detailed reports to be made with the minimum of effort. On the back of each prescription pad is a yellow reminder: 'Adverse reactions? Send your yellow cards to:– . . .' Some do; in 1975 there were 5,052 reports; by 1980 this had risen to 10,179, a quantitative improvement on the efforts of the Royal College of General Practitioners who organised a limited ADR registry in 1960 and received just seventy-five reports in four years.[31]

Dr Bill Inman, until 1980 Principle Medical Officer at the CSM, made the point that twice as much reporting does not produce twice as much information. The CSM's Annual Report for 1978 adds that, 'While the Committee greatly appreciates the co-operation of doctors, experience suggests that many suspected adverse reactions still go unreported.'[32] If it is difficult for a specialist to observe important details in a clinical trial, it is correspondingly more difficult for a general practitioner who will be dealing with a great range of patients and prescribing a wide variety of drugs. For this reason alone many ADRs go not only unreported but unnoticed.

Post-marketing surveillance has been proposed as the fine tuning for drug monitoring in Britain, and a new Drug Surveillance Research Unit has been set up at Southampton University. Although drug manufacturers have pledged £750,000 over its initial period of operation, the Unit, headed by Dr Inman, has declared itself to be totally independent.[33]

Dr Inman's team has developed a 'prescription-event' monitoring scheme.[34] Doctors are sent questionnaires asking them to record all that has happened to patients treated with selected new drugs. With this information, the Unit constructs profiles of patterns of events associated with these drugs, and may design follow-up studies if hazards are detected. Unfortunately, the system suffers from a major flaw that is likely to lead to serious underestimation of adverse drug reactions. Retrospective examination of patient notes fails to reveal most drug dangers. Consequently, the effect of this exercise may be reassurance rather than genuine assessment of risks.

Currently, when received each report of an adverse reaction is studied on behalf of the CSM by 'professional medical assessors', and if action is recommended, a report may be drawn to the attention of the Committee. In addition, all the ADR information is used to build up a computer-stored profile of each drug,[35] which may percolate through the system of the CSM to the point where action is deemed necessary. This may range from the modification of the information given in the drugs data sheet to a warning issued directly to doctors.

Data sheet modification is a negotiated agreement between the CSM and a drug company. This is very much a behind-the-scenes activity, which depends on the close relationship between the CSM and the industry. The public and the medical profession are usually unaware that anything is happening.

In more serious cases the CSM may write letters to medical journals. Dr Inman maintains that, 'On occasions these [letters] have produced a good response from the profession.'[36] Obviously this is a haphazard form of communication, and gauging a good response must be entirely subjective. Over the past twenty years these journals have published hundreds of letters from doctors who are not associated with the CSM, warning of the great risks of barbiturate sleeping pills. Although this has resulted in a massive fall in their use, millions are still prescribed every year. In 1970 about twelve million prescriptions for barbiturate hypnotics were filled; by 1979 the figure was around four million, enough for thousands of addicts. If so many letters and articles in the medical and lay press fail to convince the hard-core prescribers, the CSM's few letters will have much less effect.

The next line of attack used by the CSM seems naive. Drug manufacturers can send warning letters to doctors, after agreeing the content with the CSM. These letters will of course be mailed out in the company's envelopes, usually with a distinctive trademark; predictably they stand a good chance of being dumped unopened in a waste bin. Unlike its counterparts in Australia and the United States, the CSM does not consider that a distinctive special envelope is required for these vital warnings. In view of the known ineffectiveness of this system,[37] Dr Inman's comment that this procedure is used because the drug companies prefer to send their own warnings is apt.

The CSM can send warnings directly to doctors. There are two forms, first the 'Current Problems' discussion papers, and second the 'Adverse Reaction Series', colloquially known as 'Yellow Perils'. 'Current Problems' contains information which the CSM believes the medical profession should have; each consists of one or two sheets of paper designed with the unmistakable style and impact of a British civil service department. A typical issue will discuss perhaps six drug problems in a very academic way. Current Problems Number 4, which appeared in April 1979, included this statement on clofibrate:

> A controlled trial of clofibrate (Atromid-S, Liprinal) for the primary prevention of ischaemic heart disease (IHD) has recently been reported in 10,627 normal subjects whose cholesterol levels fell within the top third of the distribution for the population. There was a 25% reduction in the incidence of non-fatal IHD in the group treated with 1.6g clofibrate daily. The total number of deaths and the crude mortality rates were higher in the treated group than the controls; there was no conclusive evidence that this increase was due to the drug. . . .
>
> It appears that there is no place for the widespread prophylactic use of clofibrate. . . . . This conclusion, however, should not be extended to patients individually treated for disorders of lipid metabolism of which hypercholesterolaemia forms a large component and which may predispose them to an increased risk of heart disease.

Since each general practitioner or consultant will be treating each patient individually, 'Current Problems' seems to be recommending no change – a dramatically different response from the Norwegian and West German bans.

Under dire circumstances a yellow peril may be issued. It will usually have a marked effect on prescribing. But the publication of a yellow peril does not mean that the drug is to be withdrawn, unless the manufacturer chooses to do so voluntarily. It simply warns the doctor of possible dangers.

A yellow peril was produced strengthening the warning about clofibrate in August 1980. This time, there was no ambiguity. Under the heading 'Clofibrate – Mortality In Long Term Use', it said:

> The Committee on Safety of Medicines has considered the findings of a WHO co-operative trial on the use of clofibrate for the primary prevention of ischaemic heart disease. The report of this long term trial indicates that men treated with clofibrate have a significantly higher mortality rate from many causes than the appropriate control group.
>
> The attention of doctors is drawn again to the fact that clofibrate is currently indicated only in the treatment of exudative diabetic retinopathy, xanthomata and specific hyperlipoproteinaemias where appropriate investigations have been performed to define the type and severity of the abnormality. On present evidence the Committee believes that the use of clofibrate for the prevention of ischaemic heart disease should be discontinued.

Is two years from the publication of results to decisive action an appropriate response time when the CSM is confronted with such clear evidence?

If a drug were considered sufficiently dangerous, the CSM could, by advising appropriately through the proper channels, have its licence withdrawn. But this is virgin territory. The CSM has not yet felt motivated, in spite of two major drug disasters since thalidomide (practolol and asthma aerosols), to test the limits of the power of its advice.

Just as different national regulatory bodies deal differently with new drug applications, shared knowledge of adverse drug reactions is treated differently in different countries. One example concerns the antibiotic erythromycin estolate, marketed as Ilosone by Lilly and its subsidiaries world-wide. In Chapter 5, we described Lilly's campaign of 'selective detailing' of Ilosone. It is capable of causing liver disease which is sometimes so severe that emergency abdominal surgery is carried out in the belief that the pain is due to gall bladder inflammation or gallstones. Many specialists believe that the use of erythromycin estolate is unjustifiable.[38]

The British CSM reacted in June 1973, with Yellow Peril No. 10, 'Jaundice and Erythromycin Estolate'. The number of prescriptions per year in England and Wales dropped from 720,000 in 1972 to just under 400,000 in 1975 and then remained fairly constant.

The FDA included a warning about the drug in the FDA Drug Bulletin in 1974. Prescribing, however, continued at a high level, apparently because many physicians remained ignorant of the hazards. From 1973 to 1979 there were between six and eight million prescriptions per year, and reports of hepatitis to the FDA remained constant.[39] Urged in August 1979 by the Health Research Group to withdraw Ilosone's NDA approval, the FDA published a proposal for withdrawal in December 1979, which was answered in February 1980 by an 18-inch-high submission from Lilly defending the drug.[40] The debate continues, as does the high rate of prescribing and the jaundice.

The Australian Drug Evaluation Committee published their conclusions in July 1973. Erythromycin estolate was banned for adults and children over six years old. For younger children, they considered the drug might be useful but they were not going to rely on guesswork. 'Further investigation on the hepatoxic potential of the drug in this age group is being undertaken.'[41]

This is not the first time the Australian Drug Evaluation Committee has acted quickly and decisively to save lives. In the early 1960s, deaths from asthma began to rise in both Australia and Britain.[42] Until 1961 about 1,000 people died each year from asthma in England and Wales. By 1966, the figure had more than doubled. The rise corresponded with the increasing use of a new type of aerosol containing bronchodilating drugs to relieve asthma attacks. As sales of aerosols rose, so did deaths. Asthma became the most common cause of death in children between ten and fourteen years old with a seven-fold increase. Substantially more deaths were also found in other age groups.

In June 1967 the CSM acted. Yellow Peril no. 5 warned: 'A small number of reports of sudden and unexplained deaths of asthmatic patients has reached the Committee . . .' It went on to point out a 'possible link between the excessive use of aerosols by patients and the recorded increase in death from bronchial asthma. This possibility is still under investigation.' Eighteen months later, in December 1968, the aerosols were restricted to prescription sale only.

The CSM was too late for thousands of children. There were over 3,500 excess deaths among asthmatics between 1961 and 1967.[43] If a small number of these children had died in any other way there would have been immediate and sustained outcry. In Britain it was all over by 1969, no outcry, and no enquiry into the action of the CSM.

Could the CSM have acted earlier? In Australia, the Minister for Health reacted to a much smaller increase in the death rate in December 1964, and actually issued a warning to aerosol users in the press. This was followed in 1965 by a warning from the Australian Drug Evaluation Committee and there was no further increase in asthmatic deaths in that country.[44]

In Britain, acknowledged drug dangers do not necessarily lead to regulatory action. Manufacturers can withdraw their products voluntarily from the market after confidential discussions with the CSM. This procedure causes concern to officials of the WHO and of the European Committee for Proprietory Medicinal Products (CPMP). Under the international agreements a national health authority is required to give the reason for any regulatory action involving the withdrawal of authority to market a drug, either to the CPMP in the case of EEC members, or to the WHO. Since the British system does not actually involve a regulatory decision, the reporting requirements do not apply. Thus, as in the case of excessive profit refunds when the British government negotiated with Roche over Valium, British self-interest acts against the wider interests of others. This time the chain of information to those who may rely on CPMP or WHO is broken.

Unusually in these circumstances, the events that led to the withdrawal of alclofenac, an anti-inflammatory marketed by Berk Pharmaceuticals, did become known. The drug had been available in Britain for seven years when German research showed that its metabolite was mutagenic.[45] No regulatory decision was taken because voluntary withdrawal pre-empted such a move. But in this case, the head of the DHSS Medicines Division wrote to his colleagues in other EEC countries to inform them of CSM concern about the mutagenicity of alclofenac.[46] However, the medical profession was given a different story. Berk told doctors that alclofenac was withdrawn because it caused skin rashes.[47] There was no mention of possible mutations, and no follow-up.

Through international cooperation, individual regulatory bodies can share the work-load and gain the advantages of mutual experience. In 1968, numerous meetings between representatives from the twelve countries which started drug monitoring after thalidomide culminated in world-scale cooperation. The WHO Drug Monitoring Centre was started in Geneva with financial help from the United States government and a multi-disciplinary team of epidemiologists, statisticians and clinical pharmacologists. Member nations are expected not only to report regulatory decisions but also to communicate their drug experience to computerised storage and analysis facilities, from which the available information becomes generally accessible to nations requiring it.

The WHO has also been working towards limited standardisation of new drug applications. The countries involved include Canada, Australia, Sweden and Britain. At the same time, the EEC is working towards common approval procedures for Europe.

The more purposeful multinational drug industry is able to exploit the many differences between national regulatory agencies. One way is via the 'domino effect' in approvals. If the FDA, for example, accepts a drug then less rigorous agencies will be inclined to do the same. It is in the drug industry's interests to give the regulatory bodies an inflated reputation for toughness. The maintenance of these reputations will mean that a drug approval almost anywhere can be used to bring pressure on other agencies for similar approval.

Differences that are not to the industry's advantage on the other hand become the subject of critical campaigns. The FDA may take a comparatively long time before allowing a particular drug onto the American market, and this relative discrepancy has enabled the industry and its acolytes to criticise the FDA for causing 'drug lag'.

Drug lag has become a highly emotive issue. The argument is that because the FDA is slow in approving new drugs, Americans are deprived of valuable, perhaps life-saving, therapy which is available to others. The main proponent of this theory is Dr William Wardell of the Center for the Study of Drug Development. In a 1978 paper[48] he claims to have shown that the number of entirely new drugs approved has declined with the increase in time taken to approve them. Examination of the way Wardell chooses his data in our view renders his study inconclusive. Nevertheless it is used as a source of anti-regulatory pressure by the industry.

Academics from other fields have offered opinions on the issue. Milton Friedman, a University of Chicago economist, has added to the tumult. In *Newsweek* magazine[49] he asserted that:

> The 1962 amendments to the Food, Drugs, and Cosmetic Act should be repealed. They are doing vastly more harm than good. To comply with them, FDA officials must condemn innocent people to death . . . Shocking it is – but that does not keep it from also being correct . . .

Senator Nelson commented to the United States Senate Committee of Small Business, 'It would have been helpful if Mr Friedman had supplied some examples – even one example – to support his sweeping charges.' The FDA asnwered with the assurance that 'no Americans are being condemned to death or misery because important drugs are being held up. There are no miracle drugs available in other countries that are not available here.'

But Milton Friedman had a ready answer to that 'bureaucratic conditioned reflex . . . Many new drugs,' he protested, 'are available abroad that are not available here – practolol and oxprenolol, to mention just two important in cardiology.'[50]

The consumer criticism of regulatory agencies is that they do not provide protection. Despite idiosyncratic success in America with thalidomide and practolol, and many other instances of regulatory success over individual hazards, protection will always be a matter of degree.

Regulatory agencies cannot protect from the unforeseen major hazard; the best that can be hoped for is that they can limit the spread by prompt recognition and decisive action.

Nor can they offer a solution for the insidious large-scale iatrogenic effects discussed in the last chapter. The systems on which they depend are not sufficiently finely tuned to extract their incidence from the general background of sickness and mortality. Predominantly regulatory agencies will operate in the safe well-tramped middle ground, where they expend disproportionately large resources for comparatively small gains.

An example is the work of Dr Cahal for the DHSS in monitoring the effects of addictive drugs in Britain. He believes that there may be thousands of people addicted to dextropropoxyphene (the main ingredient of the popular pain-killers Distalgesic, Dolasan, Darvon and others). The drug's lethal effects in overdose are well documented, and it is no more effective than safer alternatives. Yet while there is concern about the drug, there is a marked reluctance to increase bureaucratic controls on its use. The effects are distinct enough to be noticed, but not tragic enough to prompt action.

A drug hazard has to approach major and visible proportions before action is taken. But there is obfuscation well before any point of decision is reached. Information input is seriously deficient when the vast majority of adverse drug reactions fail to be reported.

Inevitably criticism of the operation of regulatory bodies returns to the source of their data: physicians. At the interface between patients and drugs they occupy the key point in the recognition of emerging drug dangers; yet they are the acknowledged under-reporters of adverse effects. Dr Inman, while at the CSM, ascribed this failure to seven deadly sins: fear of litigation, guilt, complacency, ambition, ignorance, diffidence and laziness.[51]

Even where the reporting of adverse reactions is mandatory it does not solve the basic problem. Dr Sidney Wolfe wrote[52] to FDA Commissioner Dr Jere Goyan in January 1980 suggesting that criminal charges be brought against Smith, Kline & French, for alleged failure to report serious and unexpected adverse reactions to Selacryn, a mass market anti-hypertensive. The law requires the company to report such adverse reactions within fifteen days, but SKF included twelve cases of liver damage in a routine quarterly report. Wolfe argues that these problems would have led to the earlier banning of the drug had they been handled correctly. In the meantime the company set up a massive advertising campaign to promote the drug. In a subsequent meeting between the company and the FDA, forty more liver damage cases were 'found' that had also avoided being reported within the statutory time.

Such shortcomings are compounded by the combination of inadequate incoming information with ineffective outward communication. The British Yellow Peril will significantly affect the rate of prescribing of a drug, but it is a rarely used last resort. All too often, drugs of known danger and dubious worth remain available for physicians to prescribe for trivial reasons. Even when a drug is withdrawn, communication is so hit-and-miss that doctors will still attempt to prescribe it. The last known British prescription for practolol is dated 11th August 1976 – almost a year after the drug was withdrawn by ICI. Neither will the CSM use the public media, although this can save lives. Their attitude, tinged with elitism, is that 'scaremongering in the press does nobody any good, and can cause a lot of harm [by] provoking widespread and sometimes ill-informed comment which may damage the reputation of a worthwhile drug.'[53] But a commercial reputation cannot be more important than human life.

The example of Selacryn in the United States raises the issue of the scale of clinical trials. Pre-release adverse reaction information was collected from trials on only 533 people. For a drug intended for use by millions, this is obviously inadequate. It will always be impossible for national regulatory agencies to command clinical trials that will match a drug's potential international market. Recognising this, in some European countries including France and the Netherlands, the government is able to temporarily remove drugs from the market while reports of adverse reactions are followed up. This is obviously controversial because of the disruption of treatment that it causes; and this power is not available in the United States, Britain, or most other countries.

International collaboration on suitable scale is possible, as the clofibrate trial demonstrated. And this must be the model for future realistic standards of clinical trials; the gathering of objective data cannot be left to the whim of a reimbursed or retained consultant. Nor should it be gathered from 'volunteers' such as prisoners, expendable patients or unwitting victims in the third world.

Whatever the argument on questions of scale or of systems it remains a fundamental weakness that all regulatory bodies are in the position of making decisions based upon assessments of other people's assessments. As we have seen, the sources of information on NDAs are not always reliable or honest. The drug manufacturers have total control over the information that is submitted in support of the claims for their products. It comes down, at worst, to what they decide they can get away with, and that in turn may be linked to the rising cost of developing each new drug.

Even with the best possible information input regulatory decisions can be influenced by factors which are not completely objective, or which may reflect a difference in cultural or commercial background. When the results of the WHO clofibrate trial were brought to the attention of the

CSM its reaction compared to that of the West Germans was insipid. The study was considered to be inconclusive.

The closeness of the industry to the regulatory bodies frequently muffles their voices. The wealth and political expertise of the drug manufacturers effectively contributes to the lack of any real power on the part of the regulators,[54] and this hinders their ability to act independently. Regulatory bodies are left with no option but to act only when they are absolutely certain of their facts. They are unwilling to make any statement that could lead to battle between the drug manufacturers and themselves or their governments. Manufacturers have shown that they will take national governments to court if their interests are threatened. In these circumstances there is no room for open discussion or speculation: only irrefutable evidence is acceptable. This usually takes the form of a large number of avoidable deaths, or an even larger number of maimed and disabled. For without this evidence how can one be absolutely sure?

The ultimate criticism of regulatory agencies must be one which questions their very purpose. Fundamentaly they exist to regulate and control the use of drugs. It is a passive and limiting role which relies for its operation on the acceptance of the very assumptions that the drug manufacturers subscribe to. In essence there is no philosophical difference between regulator and regulated on the fundamental question of the benefits of widespread use of drugs. They are arguing about matters of degree and acceptability, not of necessity. In this they reflect the attitudes of society at large, they are cultural victims of the philosophy of medication as are we all. And as such it is almost impossible for them to protect us.

Our guardian angels have failed us, and will continue to do so without radical change.

Chapter Eight

Keep on Taking the Tablets

MARY WILKINS

Mary Wilkins lives in the South Wales valley town of Merthyr Tydfil. Like many working-class housewives and mothers, she likes to keep her terraced house spotlessly clean. Outside the street is dreary, a cul-de-sac which degenerates into rubble, with a view of a new council housing estate rising over the hill.

In 1971 Mary was a lively twenty-seven-year old, busily involved in the social life of the area. She founded and ran a young wives' group in her neighbourhood, and enjoyed the dances and outings they organised.

Then tragedy struck her family. Her brother died at forty-four of a heart attack. This was followed within a short time by the death of her father. Mary was left to nurse her heartbroken mother, in addition to coping with her four-year-old son. It all became a strain.

'I found it difficult to cope. I began to suffer with palpitations, and because of my brother's death I was afraid of heart disease. So I went to my doctor, and for five weeks he took my pulse, and then he referred me to see a consultant at the hospital.'

The consultant told Mary: 'You are a very lucky woman. We've got just the thing for you. It is a new wonder drug that has the effect of putting a brake on the heart.' He started her on practolol, brand name Eraldin.

'Now I know I just had the effects of the strain. But you can understand why I was worried. The tablets did stop my palpitations, but within three months I was having very heavy periods. It was a drastic change, and I often felt dizzy and giddy. I told my doctor, but he seemed to take no notice.

'One morning five or six months later, I went completely blind for about two hours. I was horrified and confused; it was like going into a tunnel. My neighbours called the doctor, and he looked for haemorrhage behind my eyes, but found nothing. I was prescribed tinted glasses and told to bathe my eyes with salt water.

'Then I went blind a second time a few months later. The doctor asked what tablets I was taking. I told him Eraldin and Tryptizol. He said, "Stop taking the Tryptizol".'

Already Mary's story is complex. The deaths in her family and the subsequent demands made upon her may well have caused sufficient anxiety to give her palpitations. It is quite possible that the heavy periods and the temporary blindness were also related to emotional stress. Taking her off Tryptizol, an antidepressant, in response to her sudden blindness, would seem to be something of an irrational reaction, though not questioning her practolol therapy is more understandable.

Practolol is a beta-blocker. Beta-blocking drugs should never be withdrawn abruptly because this can lead to a rebound worsening of symptoms and disturbances of heart rhythm which can be fatal.

'By 1973 I had deteriorated an awful lot. I started keeping a diary. It was something I had been told to do when my son Simon was ill, to see if a pattern emerged. I was still suffering with my eyes; the specialist told me it was migraine, but I know I never had migraine.

'Gradually it got so that I was in constant pain. I know it sounds ridiculous, but I was aching all over, like having 'flu all the time. My doctor handed me continual prescriptions for pain-killers.

'Then I developed a severe pain in my neck. I could not get up or move for three days. I was sent to Casualty, where they X-rayed me, but they couldn't find anything broken. The doctor asked me if I'd been in a car accident. I said no, but he insisted that I must have been in a car crash, because I had a whiplash injury to my neck. He prescribed a surgical collar, and another kind of pain-killer. I was told to keep on taking the tablets.

'After a while I was able to get about with the surgical collar, and the pain died down. But I was frightened; there seemed to be so many things going wrong. I was still wearing tinted glasses because my eyes hurt; my ears ached; they were noisy and ringing. And my skin was itchy. I cried a lot and was very depressed; nothing the doctors did seemed to make anything better, it just seemed to get worse. And by this time I knew that the doctors had put that neat little label on me – neurotic.

'By the middle of 1974 it was very rare for me to sleep, although I was prescribed several different sleeping pills. The pain had become too great. I had stomach trouble and an itchy skin, my nose and throat were so sore and dry. I used to drip water down my nose to try to ease it. At the time it seemed slightly crazy, but I have since met other Eraldin victims who have done the same.'

In November 1974 Mary broke into a rash and began to have severe stomach pains. Her chest tightened and she had difficulty breathing. When her GP called, he told her to stop taking Eraldin immediately.

'You are suffering from side-effects,' he told her.

Later, the hospital consultant strongly disagreed. 'There is nothing wrong with Eraldin,' he told her. 'You should keep on taking the tablets.' She refused. The rash cleared up but the other symptoms remained.

All the problems Mary described could have been recognised as the result of her adverse reaction to practolol. The classic practolol syndrome includes a skin rash, eye problems, tinnitus and ear pain.[1] Changes in the membrane of the throat were recognised in 1974,[2] and joint pain and neck problems had been described in the *British Medical Journal* as adverse effects of practolol in 1973.[3]

Discovering the cause of her problems did not mean they were solved. Practolol has long-term effects. By 1976, Mary had lost more than two stone in weight; yet her stomach was huge – not a development that would pass without notice and comment in the close communities of South Wales. And as frequently happens, the gossip had a painful edge.

Mary's son Simon came running in to her in tears. 'Mummy, are you going to have another baby?' Her assurance that she was not only increased his tears and distress. Becoming finally a little calmer, he told her what the neighbours were saying: 'Either she's going to have a baby, or she's got cancer.' Mary was left shuddering with tears and feeling very sick.

In her GP's opinion she was pregnant; but Mary was emphatic that this was not possible. She was referred to the hospital where she had a hysterectomy, and a mass of fibrous tissue 'like a big grapefruit' was removed from her abdomen. It was not cancer.

The painful after-effects of practolol continued all over her body. Her husband began to despair. In addition to sleeping pills, painkillers and tranquillizers, Mary was now given tablets for her vertigo. She was walking into things and falling over. 'How can you possibly have all these things wrong with you?' her husband asked. Their relationship was becoming strained.

In spite of all this, Mary took a job; but this failed because she kept falling over. In 1978 she had to have another operation, this time to cauterise scar tissue and remove polyps. After she had recovered from this, Mary decided to see another consultant privately; she was frightened of the man who had tried to make her continue to take Eraldin, and felt that he was so unsympathetic that he would do nothing to help her.

She was admitted to hospital for six weeks of extensive tests. Sixteen doctors, including a neurologist, examined her. All the tests – EEG, lumbar punctures, specific tests for various diseases – proved negative. No brain tumour, no signs of stroke, no signs that would fit an established diagnostic pattern. Mary recalls, 'I felt awful, just as if I had been poisoned. And I was treated like a thing, nobody every talked to me as if I was a person. I asked lots of questions – after all, it was me, my body they were dealing with – but they tended to ingore me, and you don't feel so clever with no clothes on . . . I just pretended not to be interested after a while, and tried to listen to what they were saying to each other about me. Once I heard one doctor say to another while they looked at my notes, "Can you see what she's been taking? Be careful what you say." And the neurologist from Cardiff seemed angry: "Why do you put young women on beta-blockers for all these years?" he asked. He wanted to know if I had any side-effects, but they told him I hadn't.

'Just before I left the hospital, the consultant said he would come and sit and chat with me and explain what had been going on. I felt so happy and relieved! But when the day came, he walked right by my bed. I cried out to him, but he refused to discuss it. I felt that black horror coming over me and just cried. The Sister said he would see me in Outpatients, but he never did.'

Mary was discharged from hospital a very sick and unhappy woman. She was told to go and see her GP; he, with another member of the practice present, was to give her a message from the consultant. 'First,' he told her, 'The good news. Your problems have nothing whatsoever to do with Eraldin.' Mary was incredulous. 'Now the bad news,' the doctor continued. 'The consultant has diagnosed multiple sclerosis.'

It is impossible to describe Mary's feelings on hearing this. She was taken home in a state of shock. Yet with characteristic resilience, it was not long before she had joined the local Multiple Sclerosis Group. 'They are very brave people, and they were very kind to me. But I knew I wasn't one of them. My symptoms are entirely different from theirs. My balance problems are in my head and neck; theirs are in their limbs.' It was subsequently confirmed that Mary was not suffering from multiple sclerosis.

Mary cannot stand unaided and she has to use a walking frame. She can sit in a chair, although she has to wear a surgical collar all the time. The determination and strength which carried her through the horrifying experiences following her period on Eraldin have surfaced in her involvement in the Eraldin Action Group. Mary's main concern is that her story should be told, and that the right conclusions should be drawn from her experience. 'I don't know what will happen next. I live from day to day, and I still have this terrible feeling that I have been poisoned. You know the worst thing? My son has never seen me well. I started a young wives' group here, years ago. But when you can't dance any more, they don't want to know you.'

In retrospect, it is astonishing that so many doctors who treated Mary Wilkins were so adamant that she was showing no adverse reactions to practolol. Systemic Lupus Erythematosus (SLE) is a complicated syndrome which was recognised as an adverse effect of practolol by the cardiologist, E.B. Raftery. It is an auto-immune disease which can be set off by a range of causes, but practolol caused it particularly often. It seems that the drug somehow leads the body to reject its own tissues as foreign. Raftery's descriptions of cases, published in the *British Medical Journal* in 1973,[4] include many of the same symptoms as Mary experienced, particularly neck and joint pains. Raftery's patients did not recover completely after practolol was withdrawn, but needed special treatment for a year afterwards; even then, they were not completely normal.

Ear problems, photophobia (inability to tolerate bright light) and skin rashes are also frequent effects of practolol; and the development of fibrous tissue in the abdomen is recognised as one of its most serious hazards. Nevertheless, Mary's doctors decided – as she realised – that she was neurotic and not a victim of the practolol syndrome. It is an all too common reaction.

SUSAN JAMES

Skin rashes are the most common drug reactions,[5] and at first they may appear trivial. But this is not so; a skin reaction can be the first sign of a process which could end in death; and some types are in themselves extremely unpleasant for the sufferer.

Susan James of Walsall took Eraldin. In 1976, she wrote: 'Like the other people, I was treated for angina, and put on the Blue Pills about four or five years ago. At first it was two pills a day, then three. About three years ago my hands started to dry up. I tried to cure them myself but each day they got worse; the pain was unbelievable. My doctor said it was a form of dermatitis, but treatment for this did no good. Another doctor treated me, he tried everything to no avail. No one had ever seen hands like it.

'Flesh was peeling off and they kept bleeding. Every little line on my hands and fingers split open. I cried and cried. Some nights I never went to bed.

'My finger nails grew hard, thick and yellow. I had to file them, they were like stone, and I wore coverings for my hands day and night. It was a nightmare that lasted about twelve months and then they gradually started to heal. Then my eyes started smarting and drying up. I thought I must have touched them with my fingers, and I started bathing them, bought eye lotions, but they got worse. The doctor gave me eye lotions and antibiotics. By this time I thought I was going mad . . .'

The story becomes the now familiar relentless one of more and more problems. Mrs James was told by her optician that she had a blood condition. Her eyes began to discharge and her sight was clouded, so badly at times that she was, to all practical purposes, blind. The sun and strong light hurt her eyes. Then she began to suffer from stomach pains and vomiting. Her ears began to ring and ache.

None of the treatments prescribed for these various afflictions had any beneficial effect. Predictably, she was told to keep on taking the tablets until one day:

'It was about May or June 1975 that the doctor's receptionist told me that the tablets had side effects and I could not have any more. My doctor clearly did not know. Another doctor took one look at my eyes and said, yes, it was the tablets.'

Mrs James's doctors were very guarded. All her other illnesses they firmly attributed to her age; she was sixty-three. 'I saw a consultant at the hospital for blood, heart, lung and urine tests. After this I had notice to find another doctor. It would appear I was wasting my own doctor's time. He said he did not seem to be doing me any good.'

Part of the problem with some drug reactions is that the victims tend to be older people who may be suffering similar symptoms as a natural part of the ageing process. This is particularly true of practolol, where, as the cases quoted show, the syndrome associated with the drug crept on insidiously over a number of years.

But there have been numerous younger people on these long-term drug therapies. Ann Jones was one.

ANN JONES

Like Mary Wilkins, Ann Jones is Welsh, and her story is traumatic. A pretty, intelligent girl, she was married and had three children by the time she was twenty-two. In 1972 she was in hospital for a routine womb operation when the surgeon accidentally perforated her uterus. Ann went into shock. As she recovered, her heart rate and blood pressure were far too high, and only Eraldin seemed to be effective.

In the next three and a half years she took more than 8,000 Eraldin tablets. During that time, the relentless story began to unfold. She made four visits to eye specialists, six visits to ear, nose and throat specialists, five visits to a gastro-enterologist, two visits to a psychiatrist, five to heart specialists, one to a neurologist, and in addition had a number of consultations with gynaecologists.

In 1977, Ann was able to take stock of her situation after five years. She wrote:

'My eyesight is extremely poor in the sense that I suffer constant double vision and visual disturbance similar to those caused by migraine. My hearing is also impaired and I have been told by a specialist that I suffer from low tone deafness. I have frequent ringing in my ears and loss of balance.

'I experience constant pain in all my limbs and in my abdomen and have been prescribed pain-killing drugs continuously since the symptoms appeared. My other complaints have included severe depression and skin rashes and numbness in my right side. I also frequently suffer from nausea and vomiting and in five years these have shown no sign of abating.

'The heart condition for which I was originally treated returned in less severe form when Eraldin treatment was withdrawn, and has remained much the same ever since.

'I have no idea what to expect from the future, nor any assurance that my eyesight or hearing will improve, or even remain as they are.

'I feel that my health is so seriously impaired that I cannot look forward to leading a normal life. On many occasions I have become convinced that I am dying.'

Behind this calm appraisal hides five years of growing fear and horror, of waking to new pain, of anxiety that she might be going mad. And the reaction of those to whom she looked for help confirmed her apprehension. In letters to Jean Trainor of the Eraldin Action Group, Ann said: '. . . In my own case I am finding it extremely difficult to get help, or even admission of the cause of my illness. Please will you give me help or advice? The doctors seem to be obstructive, or vague, and really at one time I thought I was going mad and imagining it all.'

Ann's husband heard about the Eraldin Action Group on the Jimmy Young Show on BBC Radio; but although bringing sympathy and understanding, the Action Group could do nothing to halt her personal tragedy. Her husband left her; and as at this time she was suffering from the same neck and spinal injuries that were later duplicated in Mary Wilkins, her children were taken into care.

'I am only 27 now, and for the past five years life has barely been worth living. I have three young children and I want to be happy and healthy for their sake, as well as my own. Not enough is being done for Eraldin victims. I know ICI acted in good faith, and so did the doctors, but surely we are entitled to help now, and research into making us better?'

We cannot finish Ann's story. We can tell you she became more depressed, and was admitted as a voluntary patient into a psychiatric hospital. In the hospital her intelligence and courage impressed the staff. But for Ann there was no answer in their care; she discharged herself and disappeared.

Practolol was first synthesised in ICI's laboratories in July 1964.[6] The pharmaceuticals division of the company specialises in drugs to control cardiovascular conditions, and it was claimed that practolol offered considerable advantages over propranolol, the other available beta-blocker. It was thought to be more specific in its action, and lacked some disadvantages, especially for asthmatic patients.

In July 1966 ICI made its first formal submission for practolol to the CSM. The one volume document was accompanied by a letter which made a proposal for a clinical trial, and although the toxicity data were judged inadequate, the CSM replied in September that they had no objection to a pilot clinical assessment. But they added as a rider: 'Before a full scale trial is undertaken, the Committee would require to be provided with more adequate toxicity data, and they would also wish to see the results from the investigations.' At this stage ICI had tested for acute toxicity in rats and mice. To test for prolonged toxicity, ICI gave the drug to rats and monkeys for two weeks.

ICI made their second submission in October 1967, and accompanied it with a proposal to extend the clinical trials to oral medication. The prolonged toxicity tests had been extended to include the administration of practolol to 70 rats and 24 dogs for a period of thirteen weeks. ICI felt able to conclude that: 'ICI 50,172 (their reference number for the drug) is remarkably free from toxic effects. We have observed no changes which we think would contra-indicate its administration to man at the advised doses.' Five years after thalidomide the CSM seems suddenly to have remembered the episode which had brought it into being, and in November refused to agree to the proposed clinical trial in the absence of 'full teratogenicity tests'.

After careful consideration of evidence submitted by ICI in March 1968 on three groups of thirteen pregnant rabbits which had been given practolol from conception to the twenty-eighth day of pregnancy, the Committee was able to state within twenty-four hours that there was now no objection to the proposed clinical trial.

The third submission made by ICI in January 1970 was in six volumes. It contained further long-term toxicity tests (100 mice had been given practolol for eighteen months) and it reported on the clinical trials with humans. The document nicely differentiates between 'volunteers' and 'patients' among the 900 people involved. One of the latter was given over twelve times the normal dose of the drug, 4000 mg per day. One result of the pharmacological assault was abnormal liver function. Next, 127 other patients were given practolol for periods varying between four and eighteen months, with no serious adverse reactions; indeed the most tangible side-effect to emerge from the trials appears to have been constipation.

A conference sponsored by ICI was held on 5th and 6th June in London at the Royal College of Physicians, on 'Advances in Adrenergic Beta-receptor Therapy'. Papers were read on all aspects of practolol to the sixty-six doctors who attended, three of them from ICI. On 26th June the CSM stated that they had no objection to the marketing of practolol, and on 29th June 1970, Eraldin was released on the British market.

Sales went well, and the number of prescriptions for practolol in the UK rose dramatically. In 1972, 501,700 were issued and in 1974, 898,200. The drug was also exported and widely used in other countries. A letter published in the *Lancet* in May 1972[7] detailing a reversible severe skin rash in a seventy-five-year-old patient passed without comment in the medical press. By January 1974, twenty-one such cases had been recorded, and the information included in the drug's data sheet. Then in May that year the *British Medical Journal* published a letter from Drs Felix and Ive,[8] describing a new development, a distinctive, but apparently reversible, psoriasiform eruption of the skin. There was no suggestion that any other part of the body was involved. At this time the CSM had received only one yellow card on practolol.

After the drug had been in use for four years, the practolol syndrome began to emerge. In June 1974 the *BMJ* published a letter from Mr Peter Wright[9] of London's Moorfields Eye Hospital associating practolol with damage to the front of the eye, particularly the tear ducts, which resulted in dry eyes. When ICI followed this up a month later it was obvious that a new and serious reaction had emerged, and on 10th July they informed the CSM of this development.

Two days later a draft letter was agreed between ICI and the CSM. It was to be sent by ICI to all doctors informing them of the danger of eye lesions. ICI marked the envelopes 'IMPORTANT – NOT A CIRCULAR', which in a more innocent age might have been accepted but in 1974, when printed alongside ICI's trademark, could easily have meant that the envelope went unopened by many doctors. As the reports of serious reactions rose, and claims for damages began, ICI sent a further letter in October. These letters, and various articles in medical journals, had no detectable effect; practolol prescribing continued to increase. Detailed study of prescribing by a representative sample of general practitioners from September 1974 to July 1975 confirms this rise, and the absence of effect of ICI's actions.[10]

By October 1974 the elements of the full practolol syndrome had emerged. Of the 164 ADRs on record at that time, the majority of patients had dry eyes and skin eruptions, but the remainder showed hearing problems, pericarditis, and sclerosing peritonitis.

In November ICI's Legal Department reported to the Pharmaceuticals Division. After stating the steps that the company must take to protect itself it concluded that, having regard to the circumstances at that time,

ICI were not obliged to withdraw practolol from the market. Among these circumstances 'the fact that it was believed that no patient suffered permanent ill-effects provided that practolol was withdrawn on the appearance of the first symptoms'.[11]

Practolol qualified for the most drastic action the CSM would take in January 1975. To illustrate the tone and scope of a 'yellow peril' in full cry, we quote from No. 11, 'Practolol and Ocular Damage':

> By the end of 1974, 187 reports had been received of adverse effects on the eye occurring in patients who have been treated with practolol ('Eraldin'). Two-thirds of these reports described diminished tear secretion and conjunctivitis, and the remainder, corneal damage leading on occasion to impairment or loss of vision. These effects on the eye have been noted in patients who have received practolol for periods ranging from a few weeks to several years.
>
> There are also several hundred reports of psoriasiform or hyper-keratotic skin reactions and 25 patients have complained of deafness. Fourteen patients have developed a syndrome resembling lupus erythematosus and 8 have developed an unusual form of sclerosing peritonitis.
>
> Half the patients with eye changes had a rash and in others these adverse reactions were multiple. The mild eye changes and the majority of skin reactions usually recover when practolol has been withdrawn, but the outcome with corneal involvement is less certain and the damage may be irreversible . . .
>
> In view of the serious and unusual nature of these reactions, patients who need to continue to receive long-term treatment with practolol should be carefully observed with a view to the early detection of adverse reactions.

As long as the effects were monitored, doctors remained free to pre-scribe, and ICI free to sell and promote practolol.

The yellow peril did have an immediate effect on prescribing. In February the number of prescriptions dropped dramatically, and con-tinued to do so until by July it was less than a quarter of the January figure. During this decline ICI sent out a third letter to doctors in April. It noted that 'The reactions affecting the eyes and more particularly the peritoneum have proved to have such an incidence and severity for us now to recommend that "Eraldin" should be reserved for the treatment of patients where it has specific benefit compared with alternative forms of treatment.' It was accompanied by a new data sheet which set out in detail the various reactions to practolol and described them as 'The practolol-induced syndrome'.

The full horror of the syndrome began to unfold in May 1975. In the *British Medical Journal* Drs Halley and Goodman of High Wycombe revealed[12] that one year after withdrawing practolol from a patient because of a rash, fibrosing peritonitis was diagnosed. It became obvious that withdrawal of the drug at the onset of a rash did not avoid the development of serious disorders.

ICI voluntarily withdrew practolol from use by general practitioners in the UK on 1st October, 1975, although it remained available for short-term use in hospitals in extreme circumstances. There are estimated to be 7,000 practolol victims in the UK.[13] The drug went through all the checks and safeguards set up to protect patients after the thalidomide tragedy, all the systems worked as intended; yet disaster was not avoided.

A large number of practolol victims are still alive, and some are putting pressure on ICI for compensation. But are ICI liable for the damage their drug has caused? It was approved by the CSM, and subject to their monitoring procedures in use. It was prescribed for the patients by their doctors. Who then must accept the responsibility for those damaged or even killed by a drug in these circumstances?

Doctors are not responsible, provided they act in good faith. And the CSM cannot be blamed, provided it acts within the provisions of the law. So we are left with the drug manufacturer; and the answer to the question of the company's liability must be considered in two parts. Is the manufacturer liable at *law*? That is, could you sue the company, and get damages under the provisions of the law through the courts? Is the manufacturer *morally* responsible? If so, what can, or should, be done?

ICI sought the opinion of Mr C.M. Clothier QC and Mr Peter Crawford QC to determine their precise legal responsibility. Their opinion runs to forty-six pages of record, analysis and conclusion. It states:

> The total number of patients who took the drug for substantial periods of time is not known with certainty, but it is believed to be at least 100,000 in the United Kingdom. We have been asked to consider whether any liability attaches in law to ICI to pay damages to those persons or any of them. We have separately and without consultation considered the very substantial amount of documentation. In view of the fact that this will inevitably be a lengthy Opinion we think it desirable to state our conclusion at the outset. In our opinion ICI is under no liability in law to pay damages to any person who has sustained injury in consequence of the administration of Eraldin (practolol).[14]

In their reasoning for this conclusion Clothier and Crawford lay bare the legal bones of the situation at the time of their Opinion, June 1976. The law is stark. 'A manufacturer of products . . . owes a duty to the consumer to take reasonable care.' In view of the special and particular circumstances that would apply to the manufacture and marketing of drugs, the question resolves itself to this: 'Have ICI observed the high standard of care which society is entitled to expect from a manufactuer of pharmaceuticals in these times?'[15] The conclusion was that they had.

If ICI had fulfilled the requirements of the law, what of their moral obligation? The company can be criticised for not taking the drug off the market sooner than they did, and for not advising doctors in clear and unequivocal terms against issuing further prescriptions. Moral judgement on their action in continuing to market practolol in the Caribbean, and in giving withdrawn UK stocks to poor hospitals in third world countries, will be a matter of personal opinion. In Britain they have set up a scheme to pay compensation to cases which they accept as suffering from practolol damage.

With at least twenty-one recognised symptoms of practolol damage, claim assessment is complicated. ICI have however set up a scheme with claimants' solicitors to filter the genuine from those suffering similar afflictions. Inevitably the scheme will not satisfy all claimants; inevitably the company has been accused of using delaying tactics, in the hope that some will die or tire of the process. Some conditions, such as sclerosing peritonitis, can only be positively confirmed by surgery, and many sufferers are unwilling or too enfeebled to undergo this. Whatever the criticisms, it is the opinion of the group of solicitors handling many cases that under the ICI scheme compensation is in line with what could be obtained at common law if liability were not at issue.[16]

The personal problem of being compensated for drug damage is not one of law, or liability. It is simply that the damaged and debilitated individual is alone, facing the medical establishment and the might of a large multinational corporation. Although in some parts of the world, notably those where exemplary damages will attract free initial legal assistance, the situation is changing in favour of the claimant, it still remains true that money and might have the advantage.

The situation where a person is damaged by drugs taken by his or her mother during pregnancy is irresolvable. Thalidomide is the most familiar example; but the case of the synthetic oestrogen DES, which caused a greatly increased risk of genital cancer among the children, has been noted earlier. The synthetic form of the hormone was given to mothers who were felt to be in danger of aborting, or who had a record of spontaneous abortion.

DES was found to be ineffective for the prevention of miscarriage. Additionally, since the 1950s, it had been known to cause cancer in a range of animals.[17] With the discontinuation of the use of DES during pregnancy, other synthetic hormones were marketed for the same purpose. These are progestogens, which are related to naturally occurring progesterone, and 588,000 prescriptions were written for them in 1972 in America. Like DES, progestogens were demonstrated to be ineffective for the maintenance of pregnancy, and in 1973–4 pregnancy-related indications were deleted from their labelling by the FDA.

However, this had little effect; 533,000 prescriptions were written for progestogens in 1975, despite a specific warning in the *Drug Bulletin* for January/March of that year.[18] It said: 'FDA emphasise that estrogenic and progestational hormones should not be used in early pregnancy for any purpose. Such use of these sex hormones may seriously damage the foetus (congenital anomalies, including heart and limb reduction defects) . . . no sound basis exists for use of these hormones during early pregnancy. . . .'

This warning was not echoed in the 1976 edition of the Physician's Desk Reference. In June of that year Dr Sidney Wolfe published a paper entitled 'Sex hormones used in pregnancy and birth defects: another thalidomide'. As well as pointing out the PDR omission, Wolfe cited the work of Dr Dwight Janerich of the New York State Health Department who concluded that mothers who took these drugs had five times more chance of producing deformed babies than those who did not. Since that time in America the drug has contained a patient package insert (PPI) specifically warning the consumer of this risk and advising against use during pregnancy.

In Britain, the CSM has put no such restrictions on the use of progestogen. The British edition of MIMS carried advertisements for three types of progestogen in 1973; by 1979 the number had risen to five. They are widely used for the purpose for which they have been shown to be ineffective – that is, for the prevention of spontaneous or habitual abortion. There is another way a woman might take progestogen in early pregnancy; this is by continuing to take oral contraceptives after she has become pregnant.

In 1978 the market leader was Schering's Primolut Depot, of which nearly 80,000 ampules were prescribed. In 1979 Schering withdrew Primolut Depot, and replaced it with a slightly different protestogen brand named Proluton Depot. The other progestogens available are Upjohn's Provera, Duphar's Duphaston and Organon's Gestanin. Some of these forms have alternative uses for gynaecological and menstrual problems.

The first sign that all might not be well with the offspring of mothers given progestogens were reports of virilisation of female babies. A disturbingly high proportion were born with sexual organs so grossly deformed that the clitoris looked like a penis. Then evidence began to appear in the medical journals that these babies were more likely to be born with other major malformations, including heart disease and limb deformities. In

1977 the *British Medical Journal* carried a report[19] of 104 infants with congenital heart disease, and the authors showed that exposure to sex hormones was 8.5 times more common among these babies than a matched group of normal babies. They concluded that 'controlled clinical trial should certainly be conducted to determine whether the benefit outweighs the risk'.

Progestogens have been shown to cause abnormalities known collectively as VACTERL. This comes from the parts of the body affected: Vertebral, Anal, Cardiac, Tracheal, Oesophegal, Renal and Limb. These parts of the body develop simultaneously in the foetus and if more than one such anomaly appears the cause could well be a drug. Reports of VACTERL began to appear in the 1960s when the use of oral contraceptives became widespread. The results of a five-year study of babies with three or more major VACTERL malformations were reported in the *Journal of American Medical Association* in 1978.[20] it was found that the risk of VACTERL was more than eight times greater among babies exposed to synthetic hormones, and the risk of a single major deformity was three times greater.

Inevitably in Britain and elsewhere many doctors remain ignorant of the hazards for their patients and their unborn children. Without warning or guidance from the regulatory bodies they continue to prescribe these ineffective and dangerous drugs to thousands of pregnant women every year.

JOAN DANIELS

Joan Daniels, from Mountain Ash in South Wales, was one of an estimated 8,000 women who were given Schering's Primulot Depot in 1975. Of her six previous pregnancies only one had reached full term. She had two injections of progestogen a week in the hope of avoiding another miscarriage when she became pregnant for the seventh time. In this she was successful, but all was not well and she required a Caesarian section because of the baby's distress during labour.

It was immediately obvious that the baby was unable to breathe and it proved impossible for the doctors to put a tube down his throat to help him. He was taken straight to another operating theatre. There surgeons found that his windpipe (trachea) was joined to his oesophagus, and saliva was running into his lungs. Two inches of his oesophagus were missing. The surgeon separated the pipes, and made a hole through the abdominal wall into the stomach so that the baby could be fed. On completion it became obvious that the baby still could not breathe, so he was reanaesthetised and the wound re-opened. There was another hole in his trachea.

After further surgery the baby could breathe, but for the next nine days he required continuous attention from nurses. Then yet another operation was performed to lead his oesophagus out through the side of his neck.

Joan saw her baby for the first time after this. 'I didn't know what to expect,' she said, 'I was afraid he might be a Frankenstein monster, all bits and pieces. But he looked perfectly normal wrapped in a blanket.' Fortunately, Joan loved baby Matthew immediately. Her next two years were to be devoted to feeding him through a gastrotomy tube, coping with his relentless vomiting, and nursing him through five more operations.

By the age of four, Matthew could eat and breathe through his improvised tubes. He was sick often, but although pitifully thin he had definite plans to be a footballer one day. 'I used to look at those photographs of starving children,' Joan recalled, 'and then look at Matthew with his little stick legs. If I were a worrier I'd be tearing my hair out now.' For when we met her, Joan was pregnant again, and understandably concerned about the possibility of having another deformed baby. After Matthew's birth, she and her husband had been referred to genetic counsellors, and warned that any future babies could be like Matthew although blood tests showed no abnormality in either parent. Nobody had suggested that Matthew might be a VACTERL baby, or that his problems could be linked with the use of progestogens, although the possibility had occurred to Joan. This time she had taken no drugs; we were delighted to hear that she had a healthy baby girl.

Wondering about the injections she had had during pregnancy, Joan had written to her local Community Health Council. They sought an opinion from the Community Physician, who wrote: 'The only specific risk to Primolut treatment that I have been able to discover has been the development of hermaphroditism in certain animal experiments. The risk presumably is there but has not been reported in humans. No other malformation seems to be implicated.' His letter was dated 17th August 1979. At that time information on VACTERL deformities was available, and specific details of malformations due to progestogens included in the major pharmacology reference books.[21]

The use of progestogens for threatened miscarriage has declined slightly during recent years. This probably reflects growing general disquiet about prescribing anything for pregnant women. Despite this, in 1978, over 20,000 prescriptions were issued for this purpose in Britain, and at least 7,000 babies born each year in England and Wales have been exposed to progestogens. In America a major study of over 50,000 pregnancies suggested that about 2 per cent of these babies are likely to suffer from congenital heart disease.[22] This means that around 100 extra babies will be born in England and Wales with heart defects each year because of irrational use of progestogens.

In America and Britain we can at least estimate the damage caused by these drugs. What of less fortunate countries? MIMS Africa for 1979 has thirteen separate drugs listed for use in preventing habitual abortion. These are not only progestogens, but also oestrogens and even combinations of the two. For instance, the entry for Primolut Depot, manufactured by Schering AG (Germany), starts its list of indications for use: 'Habitual abortion, threatened abortions. . . .'

If baby Matthew had been born in Africa instead of Wales he would probably have choked to death. Once the family had mourned him and buried the body that would have been that. His mother would no doubt have become pregnant again and, like so many millions of people around the world, would simply have taken on trust the medicines she believed would help.

Chapter Nine

Everyday Drug Hazards

The examples we have used of damage or death caused by drugs have occurred despite the controls and regulations instituted to prevent such tragedies. They are exceptional in that action has been taken, at least in some parts of the world, to prevent their recurrence. But the action of drugs in causing damage is far from exceptional. All potent medicines can cause adverse reactions, and such reactions are associated with the use of everyday drugs for common afflictions.

In this chapter we list some of the known adverse reactions to frequently used drugs. All the prescription medicines were prescribed in a single-brand, single-dosage form, on at least one million occasions by general practitioners in England and Wales during 1978; and this level of usage is general in most countries in the world. Most of the over-the-counter drugs described are freely available, with some national differences and restrictions. There are no figures available to indicate the quantities sold, but again we have selected the most popular types of medicines.

This is not intended to be a comprehensive catalogue or reference source, nor have we gone out of our way to select especially dangerous drugs. We have simply chosen a representative range of common medicines, most of which have value when properly used. Few adults in the Western world will not have taken at least one of the drugs at one time or another, and the majority will have experienced no particular problem. But some will recognise the symptoms they, or members of their families, developed. Comprehensive guides to medicines which can be used to check on their correct use and likely problems are available; these should be consulted whenever there is doubt or difficulty.

1   ANALGESICS

Most prescribed pain-killers are used for chronic conditions such as arthritis; predictably they are mostly taken by elderly people, sometimes for years on end. Long-term safety is therefore crucial.

Analgesics have a chequered history. The highly effective opium derivatives, now synonymous with drug addiction and overdose deaths, were freely available and thought to be harmless early this century. Opium and morphine were common components of cough mixtures and sleeping draughts. The trend in analgesics has been away from addictive opiates towards drugs related to aspirin, which has neither euphoric effects nor equivalent analgesic potency.

Many early analgesics were found wanting and have been withdrawn. One example is the dipyrone group of drugs, no longer used in most affluent countries because of their tendency to cause serious and sometimes fatal blood disease, but still promoted and extensively consumed in the third world.[1]

Toxicity continues to be a problem with analgesics. A long-term campaign against phenylbutazone (Butazolidin and other brands) has led to a reduction in its use because of the associated risk of blood disorders. Even so, over six and a half million prescriptions for Butazolidin Alka were filled in the United States in 1977.[2]

Even the newest analgesics are not trouble-free. Opren (benoxaprofen), introduced by the Lilly subsidiary, Dista UK, in October 1980, had been prescribed for about 250,000 people in Britain up to September 1981. By this time, it had been discovered that one patient in ten suffered a photo-sensitivity reaction, showing skin reactions even to the British sun. In addition, Opren has been identified as a cause of Stevens-Johnson syndrome, a serious disorder described more fully later in this chapter, and eye problems. These adverse reactions, unusual among anti-arthritic drugs, are in addition to the gastro-intestinal problems common to the class. The Committee on Safety of Medicines received about 1,900 reports of adverse reactions to Opren during this short period.[3]

1(a)   *Generic name: dextropropoxyphene (DPX)*
Major brand-names: Darvon, Distalgesic

At the end of the 1970s and continuing into the 1980s, concern about analgesic toxicity has centred around dextropropoxyphene (DPX), the major component of Distalgesic, the single most prescribed drug in the UK in 1978.

It is related to the highly addictive heroin substitute, methadone, so it is hardly surprising that it is addictive, particularly if the patient takes slightly more than the recommended dose.[4] Addiction and dependency are associated with problems of overdose, and this is the major hazard of medicines containing DPX. As little as two to three times the normal dose can be toxic. For many conditions the recommended dose is two tablets four times a day; ten or more tablets taken over a short period can be lethal, particularly if taken with alcohol.[5]

DPX causes more deaths in the United States than any other drug. Alcohol is often, but not always, involved. About a third of the one to two thousand deaths each year attributed to DPX are accidental; the other two-thirds are suicides.[6] Even the suicide figures include an accidental component, for many overdoses seem on investigation to be *cris de coeur*: unfortunately the unusual toxicity of DPX means that the help that was sought by means of deliberate overdose often comes too late. The drug can kill within half an hour,[7] with morphine-like respiratory depression. Delirium and convulsions are also common.[8]

The commonest side-effects of DPX in normal doses are dizziness, drowsiness, nausea and vomiting. Constipation, abdominal pain, weakness, headache, euphoria, insomnia and skin rashes may also occur. There have been reports of congenital malformations in children born to mothers who took DPX during pregnancy.[9] Behaviour teratogenicity has been demonstrated in animals and suspected in man.[10]

1(b) *Generic name: ibuprofen*
Brand names: Brufen, Motrin, etc.

Ibuprofen is used to reduce inflammation and pain, often over long periods. It is related to aspirin, and like other members of this family of drugs its most common side-effects are associated with its tendency to irritate the stomach lining and the gut.[11]

Deaths due to ibuprofen are usually associated with gastro-intestinal haemorrhage or with blood disorders, for example:

> A 69 year old man with a duodenal ulcer, but with no complications, developed gastro-intestinal bleeding one week after starting treatment with ibuprofen 200 mg thrice daily. Death due to multiple factors occurred two days after surgery.[12]

Ibuprofen-induced blood disorders occur only in sensitive individuals. Unfortunately there is no known way of detecting such sensitivity before a drug reaction develops, and a single episode of drug-induced blood disease makes the patient more liable to suffer from such disease in the future.[13]

Side-effects of ibuprofen are nausea, vomiting, indigestion, diarrhoea and occasionally mouth inflammation. Other adverse reactions include headache, dizziness, nervousness, oedema (water retention), skin rash, bronchospasm (constriction of the bronchial tubes), tinnitus (noises in the ears) and blurred vision.[14]

Serious cardiovascular effects including hypertension and heart problems have been found to be associated with the use of ibuprofen. Warnings about these adverse reactions have been included in the labelling of the drug in the United States since 1977.[15]

1(c) *Generic name: indomethacin*
Brand name: Indocid

Indomethacin is used in much the same way as ibuprofen. As with ibuprofen, gastric ulceration and blood disorders due to indomethacin can be fatal, for example:

> Aplastic anaemia occurred in a 67-year-old woman who took a second course of indomethacin, 75 mg daily, for 3 or 4 days; she had received 1 month's treatment a year before. Despite blood and platelet transfusions, antibiotics, and corticosteroids, the patient died of massive pulmonary bleeding and bronchopneumonia.[16]
>
> An elderly woman died 3 days after a massive haemorrhage from rectal ulceration following treatment with indomethacin suppositories, 100 mg twice daily, for about 3 weeks. She had previously developed analgesic nephropathy.[17]

Indomethacin is also believed to be capable of masking infection, activating latent infection and causing liver disease.

> Following deaths from intercurrent infections (infections arising in the course of established illness) in children treated for rheumatoid arthritis, dermatomyositis, and rheumatic fever, the FDD (Canadian Food and Drug Directorate) recommended that indomethacin should not be used for children.[18]
>
> Toxic hepatitis, possibly due to indomethacin, caused the death of a twelve year old boy who had been given 100 mg daily for rheumatoid disease.[19]

Side-effects of indomethacin include: headache and dizziness, loss of appetite, nausea and vomiting, indigestion and diarrhoea. Stomach ulcers may develop without the normal warning symptoms. Oedema (water retention), hypertension, skin rashes, hair loss, drowsiness, confusion, psychotic reactions, convulsions, ear noise and eye damage have also been reported.[20]

2 PSYCHOTROPIC DRUGS

2(a) *Benzodiazepines.   Generic   names: diazepam,   chlordiazepoxide,
oxazepam, nitrazepam, chlorazepate, lorazepam, clobazepam, medazepam and
others*
Brand names: Valium, Librium, Mogadon, Tranxene, Dalmane, etc.

The benzodiazepines are the ubiquitous tranquillizers of the Western
world. As the generic names reveal, these are the 'me-too' drugs *par
excellence.* Some are promoted as sleeping pills, others as anti-anxiety preparations. They are prescribed and taken for a huge range of ills with a
casualness unequalled by any other group of prescription drugs, partly
because of their remarkable lack of obvious toxicity.

This is not the place to discuss the potentially damaging effects on
society of a tranquillized population. The topic has been well aired in both
allegory and non-fiction. Less subtle hazards have, however, been demonstrated. These include impairment of judgement, intoxication, interference with driving and similar skills, and paradoxical aggressive
reactions. In their book, *Psychotropic Drug Side Effects,* R.I. Shader and
A. DiMascio quote the following case:

> A 42-year old mother of four children was being seen because of
> marital relationship problems. She was a relatively quiet, self-effacing
> person with a history of mild but chronic depression. As treatment
> progressed she became increasingly anxious and agitated and chlor-
> diazepoxide was prescribed. During the course of the next three weeks
> she became increasingly irritable and hostile. She got into a major
> argument resulting in a break with a sister whom she had previously
> highly respected and adored and to whom she said she owed every-
> thing. Slight transgressions by her children became major incidents
> requiring immediate and severe punishment, whereas previously she
> rarely ever chastised them. Her relationship with her husband deterior-
> ated precipitously – she refused to attend social functions with his
> business associates and their wives, voiced her condemnation of him to
> everyone who would listen, refused to make meals for him, and
> refused to have sexual relations with him, voicing how much she hated
> him. On the last night of this three-week period, her husband arrived
> home late, went to bed, and found his wife in bed sleeping with a knife
> beside her. Consultation was required, and discontinuation of the
> chlordiazepoxide was suggested. Within a week this manifestation of
> outward aggression was no longer seen and her marital relationship
> with her husband returned to the pre-chlordiazepoxide level.[21]

The doctors who treated this woman comment that 'even acts of violence such as murder and suicide have been attributed to the rage reactions induced by chlordiazepoxide and diazepam'.

Drowsiness, although often an unwelcome effect of tranquillizer use, may not be regarded as a side-effect because this aspect of the action of benzodiazepines is exploited in their use as hypnotics.

Benzodiazepines can cause dryness of the mouth, ataxia (unsteady gait) and confusion, especially in the elderly. They interact with alcohol to exaggerate intoxication. Regular use can lead to addiction and withdrawal symptoms may be extremely unpleasant, with intense anxiety, abdominal pain, cramps and sometimes convulsions.[22] Use of benzodiazepines during early pregnancy has been shown in the United States,[23] Finland,[24] and the UK[25] to be associated with an increased risk of the birth of babies with cleft lip. It is also believed to cause behavioural problems in the children of mothers who take it in mid-term.[26]

2(b) *Tricyclic antidepressants. Generic names: imipramine, amitriptyline Brand names: Tofranil, Elavil, Tryptizol and others*

The tricyclics are the group of drugs most often prescribed for depression. They are effective, but their high level of potency is associated with serious toxicity. Their overdose hazards have been mentioned earlier in the context of childhood deaths related to the use of tricyclics for bed-wetting. Depressed patients are liable to take deliberate overdoses; those who choose to consume large quantities of their antidepressant medication often perish as a result. Tragically, this can easily happen during the first few days of a course of treatment because tricyclic antidepressants have little apparent therapeutic effect for at least a week.

Death due to normal doses of tricyclic antidepressants may be caused by heart failure, blood disease, or liver damage and jaundice. Deaths have also occurred in patients taking these drugs concurrently with another type of antidepressant, monoamine oxidase inhibitors (MAOIs).

Common side-effects of tricyclic antidepressants are dry mouth, constipation which can lead to paralysis of the large intestine, urinary retention, blurred vision, palpitations and tachycardia (rapid heartbeat), nausea and vomiting, orthostatic hypotension (suddenly reduced blood pressure on standing, often resulting in blackouts), dizziness, sweating, tremor, ataxia, fatigue, convulsions, hallucinations and skin reactions. Effects on hormone systems can lead to alterations in libido, impotence, breast enlargement and discharge. Effects on the heart include disturbances of rhythm and electrical conduction, and heart attacks (myocardial infarction).[27]

2(c)   *Phenothiazines. Generic names: chlorpromazine, trifluoperazine, etc. Brand names: Largactil, Thorazine, Stelazine, etc.*

The phenothiazines are the most important members of the group of drugs also known as 'major tranquillizers' or 'neuroleptics'. They are prescribed for serious mental illness, particularly schizophrenia, and (usually in lower doses) for anxiety or any other condition where sedation is considered to be required. The phenothiazines are particularly credited with reducing the population of mental hospitals; an alternative view of their action is 'the liquid cosh' or 'chemical straitjacket'.

The phenothiazines are one of the most common pharmacological causes of agranulocytosis (loss of white blood cells). The incidence of this frequently fatal condition has been found in some studies to be as high as one in 200 patients. Liver damage is another possible consequence of phenothiazine treatment which may also be fatal; its incidence has been estimated to be between 0.2 and 5 per cent, with an average estimate of 1.4 per cent (1 in 70 patients).[28]

Side-effects of phenothiazines are extremely common and often serious. However, many schizophrenic patients are unable to communicate adequately, and any person given a high dose of a phenothiazine approaches a state of artificial hibernation where awareness is limited.

Damage to the central nervous system by phenothiazines can result in muscle trembling and rigidity (Parkinsonism). A related group of symptoms called 'tardive dyskinesias' may appear after drug treatment has ceased; they do not respond to any known therapy and can be permanent. They include involuntary movements of the mouth and lips, lip-smacking, sucking, and chewing motions, rolling and protrusion of the tongue, grotesque grimaces, blinking, and spastic facial distortions, jerking of fingers, ankles and toes, and contractions of neck and back muscles.

Hormone disturbances are common, with breast enlargement and discharge, absence of menstrual periods, impotence and ejaculatory impotence. Phenothiazines can also cause a fall in blood pressure, disorders of heart rate, drowsiness, depression, indifference, dry mouth, pallor, weakness, hypothermia, nightmares, agitation and insomnia. Effects on the skin and eyes include opacities in the lens and cornea of the eye, pigmentation of the skin and eyes, skin rashes and excessive sensitivity to sunlight.[29]

3   DRUGS ACTING ON THE HEART AND VASCULAR SYSTEM

3(a)   Beta-blockers. Generic names: propranolol, oxprenolol, etc. Brand names: Inderal, Trasicor, and others

Originally developed and prescribed for angina and cardiac dysrhythmias (disturbance of heart rhythm), the uses of beta-blockers have spread to encompass hypertension, thyroid abnormalities, anxiety and migraine.

Serious side-effects of the type found with practolol are very uncommon with other members of this drug group. Adverse effects of currently available beta-blockers include blood disorders and occasionally fatal cardiac disturbances such as congestive heart failure and heart block. Beta-blockers must never be withdrawn suddenly from a patient who has been taking them on a regular basis because of a risk of 'rebound angina' or heart attack.

The most common side-effects of beta-blockers are nausea, vomiting, diarrhoea, fatigue and dizziness. Cardiovascular effects include slowing of the heart, low blood pressure, cold extremities, abnormal contraction of the small arteries (Raynauld's phenomenon) and pins and needles (paraesthesia). Central nervous system effects include depression, hallucinations and disturbances of sleep and vision. Bronchospasm (constriction of the bronchial tubes) and skin rashes are common in susceptible individuals.[30]

Widespread use of beta-blockers is a relatively new phenomenon and the possible dangers of taking them for life are as yet unknown. However, the Boston Collaborative Drug Surveillance Program reported a 2 per cent life-threatening adverse reaction rate for hospital use. These adverse reactions generally occurred at low doses at the outset of therapy.[31]

3(b) *Cardiac glycosides. Generic names: digoxin, digitalis, etc.*
Brand names: Lanoxin, Digitaline, etc.

The cardiac glycosides increase the force of contraction of the heart. However, to be effective they must be present in the tissues at a concentration close to that at which toxic effects occur. Side-effects are therefore very common. There have been many fatalities.[32]

Of 135 patients who were taking digitalis preparations on admission to hospital, digitalis toxicity was found in 31 (23%) and possible toxicity in 8 (6%). Toxicity was associated with an increased mortality rate and incidence of advanced heart disease, renal failure, and pulmonary disease.[33]

Eleven patients developed double tachycardia in one hospital in one year. A mortality-rate of 73% was associated with failure to recognise double tachycardia as a symptom of digitalis toxicity. Three of the 4 patients whose digitalis was withdrawn at the onset of double tachycardia survived.[34]

Marked venous engorgement of the intestine with haemorrhage and oedema of the intestinal wall were found in 10 patients who died after treatment with digitalis, digoxin, or lanatoside C. Most of the patients had complained of abdominal pain and tenderness.[35]

Symptoms of digitalis poisoning include nausea, salivation, vomiting, anorexia, diarrhoea, abdominal pain, headache, facial pain, malaise, drowsiness, depression, disorientation, delirium, mental confusion, pins and needles, blurred vision, distorted colour vision, extra heartbeats, disturbances of heart rhythm, defects of conduction, and heart failure.[36]

Toxic effects . . . occurred in 27 out of 80 elderly patients being treated with maintenance doses of digoxin. Treatment was successfully withdrawn from 59 patients. It was suggested that digoxin might be withdrawn in all elderly patients except those with primary cardiac lesion.[37]

3(c)   *Generic name: methyldopa*
Brand name: Aldomet

Methyldopa is an antihypertensive drug with a wide range of adverse effects. The most serious of these are blood disorders, particularly haemolytic anaemia, which involves destruction of the red blood cells,[38] and liver damage.

Of 20 patients with liver damage due to methyldopa, most developed jaundice 3 to 16 weeks after starting treatment; the total dose did not usually exceed about 65 gm. Four patients had recurrence of jaundice after a second course of treatment. Of the 20 cases 14 presented as hepatitis syndromes, 2 as cholestasis, 2 as active chronic hepatitis, 1 as cirrhosis without clinical evidence of liver disease, and 1 as fulminant hepatic failure; the last 2 patients died.[39]

Sexual dysfunction, although a frequent consequence of treatment with methyldopa, often goes unreported: 'In 30 men taking methyldopa the incidence of failure of erection was 7% (volunteered), or 53% after specific questioning.'[40]

In hospital, the most important problem is extreme reduction of blood pressure (hypotension), which may be life-threatening. Methyldopa was found to have an 18.4 per cent adverse reaction rate and a 19 per cent failure rate.[41]

Other side-effects include drowsiness, depression, nightmares, nausea, dry mouth, stuffy nose, stomach upsets, diarrhoea, constipation, fever, dizziness and lightheadedness. Its rarer adverse effects include headache, black tongue, oedema, pancreatic disease, salivary gland inflammation, parkinsonism, skin rash, weakness, arthralgia (joint pain) and aggravation of angina of effort.[42]

3(d)   *Thiazide diuretics: Generic names: cyclopenthiazide, hydrochlorthiazide etc.*
Brand names: Navidrex, Moduretic and many others.

Diuretic drugs are used to treat high blood pressure or any disease which causes water retention; they cause increased urination. With the large output of water, salts are excreted from the body in large quantities and some of the adverse effects of diuretic drugs are directly attributable to this action. Many of the side-effects of thiazide diuretics are shared by other diuretics such as frusemide (Lasix), although there is wide variation in potency and duration of effect.[43]

Thiazide diuretics may cause nausea, dizziness, weakness, numbness, pins and needles, skin rashes, allergic reactions and sensitivity of the skin to sunlight. In susceptible people they can induce diabetes, gout and serious blood disorders.

Most diuretics cause excretion of potassium, which can be dangerous because if severe it can result in muscle weakness, constipation, loss of appetite, kidney damage and heart dysfunction. It also sensitizes the heart to digitalis and other cardiac glycosides, which may be prescribed concurrently. Potassium is therefore often included in diuretic tablets (e.g. Navidrex-K), although this practice is not recommended by experts, for example the British National Formulary. Potassium supplements given separately can cause stomach ulceration and toxicity problems due to excess potassium. Potassium poisoning can cause listlessness, confusion, weakness, paralysis, cardiac arrhythmias (disturbances of heart rhythm) and cardiac arrest. Intestinal ulcers due to potassium can be so severe as to result in perforation and haemorrhage.[44]

4 ANTIBIOTICS

The hazards of antibiotic use are not restricted to the individual patient. Environmental pollution due to rash use of antibiotics results in the development of antibiotic-resistant strains of bacteria. These are bred in centres of high antibiotic use as divergent as pig farms and the surgical wards of major hospitals. On an individual level, allergic reactions and the risk of super-infection with fungi or resistant bacteria are common to all antibiotics, although different drugs carry their own specific risks. Overuse of antibiotics is such that even adverse reactions which occur relatively rarely in proportion to the frequency of use of the drug have become commonplace. Dr Sidney Wolfe has calculated that there are probably

30,000 deaths per year due to adverse reactions to antibiotics in US hospitals alone.[45]

4(a)   *Penicillin. Generic names: penicillin V, ampicillin, amoxycillin, etc. Brand names: Crystapen, Penbritin, Amoxil, etc.*

The most common, and potentially most serious, adverse reaction to penicillin is allergic. Mild allergy may appear as skin rash, swelling of the face and throat, fever and swollen joints. A severe, sometimes fatal, reaction can occur, involving constriction of air passages and a sharp fall in blood pressure. An individual who is sensitive to a penicillin is likely to be allergic also to other related antibiotics. Apart from sensitivity problems, penicillins are extraordinarily safe drugs. Their dangers stem predominantly from gross mis-use and profligate prescribing.[46]

In the Bostol Collaborative study, Ampicillin was found to have a 19 per cent failure rate and a 10.6 per cent adverse reaction rate. Drug rashes occurred in 4.9 per cent of patients, but the authors point out that they may be missed in many cases since they are often delayed for a week after treatment.[47]

4(b)   *Tetracyclines. Generic names: tetracycline, oxytetracycline, etc. Brand names: Aureomycin, Terramycin, Tetracyn, etc.*

The tetracyclines are active against a broader spectrum of bacteria than any other antibiotic, although some are now resistant to them. Tetracyclines are only partially absorbed from the gut and enough antibiotic reaches the lower bowel to upset the normal bacterial organisms which live there. When the balance between bacteria and fungi is altered in the gut, superinfection with thrush (*Candida*) may result. Fulminating enteritis, caused by resistant bacteria, is a very serious superinfection which can lead to death, especially after abdominal surgery. Blood disorders and liver and kidney damage may also occur.[48]

> Six non-pregnant women died after receiving large doses of tetracycline by intravenous injection. At post mortem a foamy type of fatty change in the liver was evident. Death was attributed to tetracycline in 4 patients, and 2 others were considered to have died from pre-existing disease which could have been adversely affected by hepatic dysfunction.[49]
>
> Of 158 patients referred to a renal unit with acute deterioration of renal function, 48 had received treatment with tetracycline in the previous 2 weeks.[50]

Side-effects of tetracyclines are common. They include nausea, vomiting and persistant diarrhoea which is attributed to irritation of the intestine. These drugs are deposited in teeth, bones and nails, and when given in pregnancy or infancy they can interfere with bone growth. Children treated with tetracyclines can develop permanently yellowed teeth.[51]

4(c)   *Sulphonamides. Generic name: co-trixomazole.*
Brand names: Septrin, Bactrim, etc.

Co-trixomazole is the most recently developed and extensively used sulphonamide-containing drug. It is prescribed particularly for chronic bronchitis and urinary tract infections. Both these conditions often require long-term medication, which is unfortunate in view of the fact that adverse effects of sulphonamides are more likely to occur with prolonged use. Under the Swedish drug-damage scheme, compensation is most often paid to victims of adverse reactions to this group of drugs.[52]

Sulphonamides can cause blood disorders resulting from damage to blood cells, pigment, and bone marrow. Liver damage may also be fatal; it usually occurs within three days of commencing treatment. Sulphonamides can cause severe, sometimes fatal, skin reactions such as epidermal necrosis and a disorder characterised by extensive skin lesions and mouth ulcers known as erythema multiforme or Stevens-Johnson syndrome.[53]

> Reports were collected of 116 cases (81 from the United States) of Stevens-Johnson syndrome associated with sulphonamides between 1957 and 1965. There were 79 cases in children under 15 years of age, with 20 deaths, and 37 in adults with 9 deaths.[54]
>
> From a survey of the published literature and reports to one of the manufacturers it was clear that all types of reactions to sulphonamides had been reported within 30 months of the introduction of co-trixomazole. Three quarters of all side effects were related to skin or to the gastro-intestinal tract and included glossitis and stomatitis (tongue and mouth inflammation). Rashes appeared more often in older patients, possibly because of wider use in these patients and included 6 cases of erythema multiforme and 5 (3 fatal) of epidermal necrosis. The reported incidence of rashes ranged from 1.6 to 8%.[55]

Crystals of the drug may be formed in the kidney, leading to pain, inability to urinate, or blood in the urine. Other side-effects include nausea, anorexia, fever, drowsiness, headache, mental depression, aching joints, and artery damage in allergic patients.[56]

5 ANTI—INFLAMMATORY SKIN CREAM

Generic names: betamethasone valerate, hydrocortisone, etc.
Brand names: Betnovate, Adcortyl, etc.

Skin creams prescribed for inflammation, soreness, swelling and irritation are likely to contain corticosteroids, synthetic forms of hormones produced by the adrenal glands. They mask the symptoms of infection. Often they seem marvellously effective but their long-term use entails hazards both through local effects at the site of application and through absorption into the general circulation.

When inflammation is reduced, secondary infection is more likely to occur, especially when corticosteroid cream is used under a waterproof dressing. Boils, thrush and other infections can develop. Continued use of corticosteroids may produce wasting of deep layers of the skin, producing a depressed, stripy area. Sometimes the change is permanent.[57]

> Treatment with fluorinated corticosteroid creams for pruritus and in 1 case psoriasis of the perianal area led to atrophy of the skin in 8 patients which was mistaken for the original condition. Continued treatment with the creams exacerbated the atrophy which eventually became irreversible.[58]
>
> Fluorinated steroids applied to the face could cause rosacea, perioral dermatitis, or acne. These syndromes had occurred mainly in adult women. Betamethasone valerate and fluocinolone acetonide were usually implicated. Treatment consisted of tetracycline by mouth and the exclusion of corticosteroids[59] (cf. tetracycline, above).

Corticosteroids absorbed into the system produce adverse effects including delayed wound healing and increased susceptibility to all types of infection, particularly thrush of the mouth. Eye damage can occur, and bone growth in children may be retarded whilst adult bones become porous. The effects on metabolism are too complex to describe here.[60]

6 OVER-THE-COUNTER DRUGS

Over-the-counter drugs are rarely dangerous when used as directed for short periods. There are marked variations between countries in the selection of products permitted for over-the-counter sales, but the rule is usually that those that are regarded as more dangerous are only available on prescription. Less hazardous drugs are usually also less potent: if they do little good, at least they do little harm. Unfortunately, the assumption that over-the-counter medicines are effectively harmless has led to overuse of these preparations and consequent self-inflicted illness.

Drugs available over the counter in the third world may be considerably more hazardous. Not only does the permitted range often include preparations that would not be acceptable in the better-protected rich countries,[61] but drugs officially designated 'prescription only' may be readily available from pharmacists,[62] corrupt health officials and village medicine men.[63] The distinction between prescription-only and over-the-counter drugs is often a fictitious one in these countries.

Analgesic nephropathy, kidney disease caused by excessive use of pain-killers, particularly phenacetin, is one relatively common form of illness often caused entirely by over-the-counter drugs. Bleeding from the stomach or small intestine is another. Regular doses of aspirin as small as two or three tablets a day can cause bleeding, and the daily loss of just a teaspoonful of blood can result in anaemia in time. Aspirin use in Britain is the cause of more than 7,000 hospital admissions for acute gastro-intestinal haemorrhage each year, and of six per cent of cases of anaemia.[64]

While some people take analgesics every day, with sometimes fatal consequences, others use laxatives to excess. This can lead to disruption of bowel function if continued over anything more than a short period. So-called 'health salts' are usually laxatives which are capable of producing this result.[65]

Some over-the-counter medicines are very useful; but the record of relative safety enjoyed by aspirin and paracetamol is not shared by all. Experience with the once readily-available analgesic phenacetin provides a grim warning against casual use of apparently innocuous medicines. Although phenacetin was introduced in 1887, it was not until 1953 that it was suspected of causing deaths through kidney damage. Its dangers were confirmed in a Swedish town where it was particularly popular.

In 1918, there was a world-wide epidemic of influenza. In one particular town in Sweden, the doctor at a large factory prescribed a powder containing phenacetin, phenazone (a drug related to phenacetin) and caffeine to relieve the symptoms. Those who took the powder believed that they were invigorated by it, and some continued to take it after the disease had passed, imagining that it helped them to work faster.

Use of the powder spread throughout the town. It became almost as usual to offer a powder as a cigarette. When visiting friends in hospital, a powder was 'as welcome as flowers, fruit or chocolate, whatever the nature of the illness. Attractively wrapped packets of powder were often given as birthday presents.' As far as doctors were concerned, the use of the powder was merely 'something of a joke'.[66]

The phenacetin consumption of the inhabitants was about ten times that of other comparable Swedish towns. Deaths from kidney damage rose steadily to reach three times the rate of similar towns by the 1950s.

An investigation of powder-taking was fiercely resisted by the Swedish workers. There was even organised burning of questionnaires on powder use. It was discovered, nevertheless, that the powders were taken not to combat pain but because they reduced fatigue – primarily because of the caffeine content, although there is some evidence that phenacetin can give a slight psychic 'lift'.

In 1961, phenacetin was withdrawn from sale in over-the-counter preparations in Sweden because of its record of kidney damage. The workers in the town, where the powders had been so much part of the culture, turned to a mixture of phenazone and caffeine. Sales of the powder stayed steady despite the change. Devotees claimed that 'it was quite useless, but that one had none the less to take a few now and then'.[67] Clearly, use of over-the-counter medicines is as much subject to social influences as the consumption of prescription drugs.

Even a drug with dangers as well documented as those of phenacetin may not be withdrawn for many years. In the USA at the end of 1980, the FDA had yet to ban phenacetin, and Lilly's best-selling Darvon Compound, containing both dextropropoxyphene (DPX) and phenacetin, remained available. Most companies have chosen to replace phenacetin in their products with its breakdown product, paracetamol (acetaminophen); a sound decision in view of the fact that analgesic abuse accounts for about 12 per cent of kidney failure cases, with phenacetin as the major culprit.[68]

The extent to which paracetamol is now responsible for kidney damage is uncertain. Acute overdose (as in suicide attempts) does lead to both kidney and liver damage, and prolonged use of large doses is believed to be capable of causing kidney failure.[69]

Cough and cold medicines form another group of much-used over-the-counter preparations. They generally contain a selection of ingredients of dubious efficiency, but particular pharmacological groups appear repeatedly in many different guises. These are sympathomimetics and antihistamines.

Sympathomimetics are related to adrenaline, the hormone involved in 'flight or fight' responses. They can be found in over-the-counter preparations as diverse as asthma remedies, eye drops, haemorrhoid preparations, slimming pills and cold treatments. Their main effect is constriction of small blood vessels. This leads to increased blood pressure, which is hazardous for those who suffer from hypertension or heart conditions.[70]

A 15-year-old girl who had been taking an anorectic preparation containing phenylpropanolamine 25 mg (a sympathomimetic), caffeine 25 mg, methylcellulose 25 mg and assorted vitamins in tablet form thrice daily developed transient hypertension and cardiac arrhythmias.[71]

Two young men who had taken a proprietary preparation (Contac) containing phenylpropanolamine 50 mg for acute rhinitis [runny nose] were found to have blood pressures of about 180/110 mm Hg. Their blood pressures returned to normal the day after they stopped taking the medication.[72]

A 21-year-old man who took 150 mg of phenylpropanolamine hydrochloride (in 3 Ornade Spansules) suffered the sudden onset of diffuse abdominal pain, severe throbbing headache, and nausea associated with elevated blood pressure of 240/120 mm Hg.[73]

Adverse effects of sympathomimetic drugs include giddiness, headache, nausea, vomiting, sweating, thirst, palpitations, difficulty in passing urine, weakness, trembling, anxiety, restlessness and insomnia. Some people are so sensitive to them that they exhibit these symptoms with normal therapeutic doses.[74]

Antihistamines are commonly found in over-the-counter cough and cold remedies, although there is no evidence that they have the slightest value in treating these conditions.[75] They are effective treatments for allergic reactions and are sometimes taken as sedatives.

Sedation is experienced to some degree by all who take antihistamines by mouth. It may vary from slight drowsiness to deep sleep and includes inability to concentrate, lassitude, dizziness, low blood pressure, muscular weakness and incoordination. Other side-effects include nausea, vomiting, diarrhoea or constipation, colic, stomach-ache, headache, blurred vision, tinnitus, elation or depression, irritability, nightmares, anorexia, difficulty with urination, dry mouth, tight chest, and tingling, weakness and heaviness of the hands.

Antihistamines are often given to children to induce sleep. They can act as stimulants, and overdose may cause convulsions. Adults sometimes also experience stimulation, with insomnia, nervousness, increased heart rate, tremors, muscle twitching and convulsions. Antihistamines can precipitate fits in epileptics. Antihistamine creams carry a great risk of skin sensitization and eczema, but skin reactions may also occur when they are taken by mouth. The risks of antihistamines are greatest in those who drive or operate machinery because of the danger of accidents.[76]

Drug side-effects and adverse reactions must be considered in context. While an unwanted effect may, of itself, appear to be a fairly minor affliction, it should be remembered that it is an *additional* complication for a person who is already sick. Under these circumstances, a further degenerative cycle may be triggered, delaying recovery, causing permanent damage or even ending in unnecessary death.

Part Three

Doctors and Patients

Chapter Ten

What's Wrong, Doctor?

'The patterns of illness today are of three main types.

Firstly, is the burden of chronic disease whose hallmark is irreversibility, namely circulatory disorders, chronic bronchitis, obesity, arthritis, chronic alcoholism and psychiatric illness, for which at best medical management is supportive rather than curative. Secondly is the incidence of minor self-limiting disorders such as upper respiratory tract infections, allergies and manifestations of stress such as tension headaches, indigestion and anxiety states for which medical help is frequently sought and doctor-prescribed or self-prescribed medication is the rule.

Thirdly is the group of medical or surgical conditions in which timely intervention can sometimes effect a 'cure' or improvement in the quality of life. *Unfortunately this group represents the smallest proportion of doctor–patient contacts: yet it is around such successful encounters with medical technology that the bulk of medical education and public expectation is based.*'[1]

Bryan Furnass, *The Magic Bullet*

In this chapter we shall consider the institution of the medical profession, its underlying assumptions, and the forces which cumulatively act upon the physician to produce his most common response, the writing of a prescription. The key that must be grasped is that the act of prescribing by physician for patient is essentially a social act. It usually has little or nothing to do with sickness, treatment or cure.[2]

Part of the problem with the practice of medicine lies in its professional structure. A highly effective public relations exercise has continued over centuries to convince both the public and doctors themselves that the very nature of the profession is such that its actions are certain to be beneficial. Professional people, by some definitions, are altruistic, highly skilled and uniquely qualified. They possess unchallengeable expertise and experience which has been developed through years of learning and practice. The ideal member of a profession starts with a vocation, and effectively devotes a lifetime's work to the good of the community. Professional people are usually highly regarded in society, they are seen as conferring qualities of leadership and stability, of upholding the values of the community. Of none is this more true than the doctor.[3]

Sceptics ascribe entirely different characteristics to the professions and the way their members behave. From a different perspective, professional people may be portrayed as protectively monopolistic, linguistically exclusive, 'narrow specialists with narrower vision', the conservative defenders of any *status quo*.[4]

The Royal College of Physicians was incorporated by King Henry VIII in 1518, and by royal charter commanded to oversee medicine within seven miles of London. The overt function of the Royal College was to protect the public from 'the audacity of wicked men who profess medicine more for the sake of avarice . . . than good conscience'. Covertly, its primary intention was to establish a monopoly for physicians, and to suppress the competing bodies who were struggling to increase their status at the expense of the physicians. Among these bodies were the Apothecaries, shopkeepers offering diagnosis and remedies to the poorer people. They had broken away from their parent group, the Grocers, to form their own guild in 1617, and during the Great Plague of London in 1665 it was they who provided treatment for the victims, as the Physicians had fled the city with their affluent patrons. Subsequently the House of Lords frequently found it necessary to defend the Apothecaries from attacks by the Physicians, who deeply resented their continuing involvement in medical matters. Finally, in 1858, the Medical Act established a single register for all medical practitioners, with a recognised diploma or degree. The register included the physicians, surgeons (who had become much more respectable since they had severed their connection with the barbers in the eighteenth century), and the lowly apothecaries. The apothecaries were the forerunners of today's general practitioners, and their particular interest and involvement with medicines has survived.[5]

This abbreviated English history highlights both the concern of the professions with boundaries and the need for detached adjudication. The battles are still being fought today on both sides of the Atlantic. Recent suggestions that pharmacists, whose knowledge of drugs is often superior to that of physicians, should have a role in choosing drugs for patients drew this response from a representative of the medical profession:

> Our profession is reeling under attacks from virtually every quarter, but one of the most dangerous is the attempt to deny us control over our patient's therapy . . . Leaders of the American Pharmaceutical Association [have] made statements that should scare the stethoscope off every Doctor in this country . . .

The physician went on to describe proposed legislation in California which would allow a limited list of drugs to be prescribed by qualified pharmacists. In Britain the same 'unthinkable proposition' brought forth a more measured, but equally deeply felt, rejection from the British Medical Association.[6]

Today the battle is not only between those parts of the medical industry that one would expect to work as close allies, but also between established medicine and alternative forms of treatment which are denigrated or dismissed. It is regrettable that the stringent tests of effectiveness that Western medicine has demanded of such techniques as acupuncture, for instance, have rarely been applied to psychiatry, or many aspects of obstetrics.[7] Indeed it is a fundamental characteristic of the profession that, whereas the practice and dogma of others are rejected out of hand, its own are not questioned until either the evidence is completely overwhelming, or historical perspective has rendered them irrelevant.

Effective criticism has a chance only if it is made from a position of unassailable superiority. The teacher can criticise the pupil and expect notice to be taken, but the pupil who considers that his teacher is wrong is likely to be ignored, both by the teacher and those who are in charge of or in awe of the teacher. This is the reality of the power structure that maintains institutions in hierarchical societies. In medicine the power of the professional institution is based upon its control of a body of esoteric knowledge, and professionalisation is the binding of this knowledge to its market, in a way that allows the professional the maximum control over the way demands for his services are fulfilled.

This knowledge does not consist entirely of factual or technical information. Medicine has proudly maintained its claim to be both Art and Science. Because of this, medical practitioners are trusted to exercise judgement which, in questions of life and death, transcends the power of any other group. The core of this trust is the *clinical judgement* of the individual physician, which derives from the extensive clinical training which the profession requires. In return the profession confers a protected status upon the physician.

Doctors derive their high autonomy from the esoteric nature of their knowledge and experience. Once they are qualified their activities are subject to minimal supervision. Such autonomy is associated with the ideals of public service, integrity and reliability expressed by the profession. This is complemented and reinforced by the high degree of public esteem and confidence which the profession enjoys.[8]

In Britain, where the class system throws the selection process into strong contrast, it is found that of British doctors nearly 90 per cent come from non-manual backgrounds, and 80 per cent are from the minority social classes I and II, loosely classed as 'professional and intermediate', whereas only 20 per cent come from the much more numerous other classes. Significantly, 43 per cent of all British doctors have immediate relatives who are also doctors.[9] The financial burden that years of medical education imposes on the American family ensures that a similar pattern is found in the United States. The medical profession, more than any other, exhibits linear selection, or 'job inheritance', as a significant factor in the composition of its membership.

Physicians have to gain specific qualifications before they can practise. But this process is not as straightforward as it might appear. Medical schools are remarkable for the number of years required before they deem a student qualified. While it is true that a competent physician must have absorbed a massive quantity of information, it has been demonstrated by some United States medical schools that two or more years can be cut from current training without diminishing the proficiency of the students. Despite this example, and the high cost of keeping students in medical schools, two such programmes are 'in process of being scrapped, largely on evidence that is entirely subjective and despite the fact that graduates of the six year program differ in no objective way from those pursuing the eight-year route'.

Nine-year medical programmes are becoming increasingly common. Dr Carlton B. Chapman, the President of the Commonwealth Fund, illuminated the reason for this apparently illogical extension thus: 'This clearly established trend must be saying something to us. Very obviously, the retreat to the eight-year track and even longer M.D. – Ph.D. programmes, in the face of convincing evidence that for many students six years is quite adequate, suggest a *hidden agenda* of some sort.'[10]

What is the content of this hidden agenda? Why does it require students to spend so much time at medical school, and why is it so valued by faculty members? Sociological evidence points to the importance of the medical school in inducing conformity with the norms of the profession.[11] Essentially the division between the medical profession and the laity is emphasised, and this division forms part of the armouring which both makes the physician impervious to criticism and protects him from the traumata of his occupation. More obviously it maintains the exclusivity, and thus the market value, of the profession. Consequently the professionalisation process requires that medical training be increasingly stringent, more esoteric and expensive, and take much longer to complete.

It is in medical school that the developing physician learns to rely on the unitary approach to illness that is characteristic of Western culture. Six or more years in a medical school which consistently presents health, illness and treatment in terms of one particular model means that doctors are so firmly committed to it that any other way of viewing these issues become inconceivable.

The medical model is built on concepts which are familiar to us all. A patient has *symptoms* which are caused by a specific *disease*. He consults a doctor who questions and examines him. Using this information, the doctor produces a *diagnosis*. On the basis of the diagnosis, *treatment* is *prescribed*. The patient takes the treatment *as directed* by the doctor in order to obtain the maximum benefit.[12]

The original assumption was that there was a single cause for each illness. If the cause, be it bacterium or poison, were eliminated, the illness would disappear. The germ theory, which provided the background to the 'magic bullet' concept of chemotherapy, remains dominant.[13] It is an attractive theory; germs can be seen under the microscope and grown in suitable cultures, and these micro-organisms are capable of disrupting body processes. Individuals who have been overwhelmed by germs suffer the disease these cause.

The medical model has been adapted to embrace disease with multiple causes but it still associates specific interacting causes with defined effects. Accumulating evidence of the social and psychological causes of illness have put severe strains on this limited adaptation. The medical model can only accomodate the facts of disease by becoming so vague as to be meaningless. It is also unable to account for the fact that some groups of people are more susceptible to illness of all kinds than others. Sociologist Jake Najman has demonstrated this curious phenomenon clearly by studying death rates in different occupational groups. He found that death rates from all causes varied in a way that could not be attributed to chance.[14]

Some known occupational hazards can be related to characteristics of the work, and therefore can be explained in terms of a conventional medical model. It is accepted that miners and seamen, for example, run a high risk of fatal accidents. But they are also more likely than almost any others to die early from cancers, vehicle accidents and heart disease. Tailors, bus drivers and builders share this tendency to an early death from a wide range of causes. At the opposite end of the mortality spectrum are metal tradesmen, farmworkers, technicians, company directors and, conveniently, undertakers. These groups show remarkable freedom from death from causes as divergent as stroke, cancer and accidents.

Religious groups also tend to be longer lived than the faithless, officers live longer than their men, higher social classes are healthier than lower. How can the medical model of disease, on which treatment is based, cope with these differences which depend on social, cultural and economic factors?

Medical training ignores these realities of illness. It also under-educates doctors in the use of the major tool they are given to treat their patients.

Pharmacology is usually taught in the student physician's first year in medical school. Illogically, it is introduced as a pre-clinical subject, before the student has had any practical hospital experience. Much of it is bound to be forgotten by the time the physician emerges to practise on his own patients, and what is remembered will by then be out of date.

Further training in pharmacology is almost absent from postgraduate courses for doctors, and new developments are usually presented to the physician in the form of promotional material from drug manufacturers. It is clearly very difficult for the individual physican to make an informed rational evaluation of their claims, despite all the years of training. Many general practitioners feel that their knowledge of drugs is inadequate, and that they need further training. In Britain these doctors tend to be profligate prescribers.[15]

In the United States the Network for Continuing Medical Education conducted a test designed to measure the level of knowledge about antibiotics among physicians. Analysis of the first 4,513 responses to the test showed that the majority displayed a potentially dangerous degree of ignorance, and those physicians who saw the most patients per day had the lowest scores.[16]

This may be a reflection of the fact that in 1978 only about half of the 123 United States medical schools had clinical pharmacologists on their faculties. Even more disturbing is the statement of Dr K.D. Helmon, head of clinical pharmacology at University of California Medical Center, given before a Senate Committee in 1974. Dr Helmon testified that *fewer than 10 per cent* of medical schools had courses in drug therapeutics, and although drug therapy is the most common form of medical treatment, the average doctor receives *only six to ten hours of training in pharmacology.*[17]

If medical training has been shown to be inadequate in the doctors' major area of activity, and the more practical skills can be picked up fairly quickly as wartime para-medic training shows, what then are the predominant effects of many years in medical school on the carefully selected students?

Conrad Harris has examined the impact of medical training on the personalities of students. He found that it tended to repress the intuitive and creative sides of personality, and to change the capacity for theorising into a more practical, mechanical approach. This is a classic path to conformity. In parallel, he found that medical school, more than any other form of higher education, tended to isolate the student. These processes measurably effect the performance of students in activities which might be considered crucial to the success of their function as physicians.[18]

It is catastrophic that medical education interferes with students' ability to elicit problems from patients. Their capacity for dealing with the personal problems they are bound to encounter is hobbled by an apparent loathing for direct questions compounded by a retreat into the safety of professional jargon.

A videotape study of sixty medical students at the University of Colorado demonstrated their bedside manner with simulated patients. The students were found to have developed interview techniques which hampered the collection of relevant information. They displayed a narrow focus and failed consistently to offer feedback or reassurance to their patients. Senior students were considerably worse than freshmen. The study concludes that medical school training makes communication between doctor and patient poorer.

Final-year medical students usually believe that they can empathise with patients, and that patients are favourably impressed by them. Neither assumption is justified. Their empathetic abilities are as poor as in first-year students, and patients like them less.[19]

Just as medical students avoid giving feedback to patients, doctors in general practice characteristically fail to share information with their patients. The reasons offered for this reluctance have sometimes been found to be related to the professional's belief that he does not need to be held accountable for his behaviour to his clients. In one study of general practitioners, some doctors said that they considered that it would be too boring to share details of common ailments with patients time and again. Others argued that information was potentially harmful, it could make patients anxious. These attitudes are learnt during clinical training, when consultants are notorious for their unwillingness to give information to patients.[20]

The over-simplified reticence of the professional may be particularly unfortunate for patients. It has been experimentally demonstrated that information itself can have a positive value for patients. Those who are given more information, and helped to understand their condition, have a better recovery rate and feel significantly less pain than those left in the dark.[21]

Western medical schools have evolved a training regime that is designed to fit students for their future role as medical professionals. But balance is lacking. Their skills and virtues appear to be invested more in an inward-looking maintenance of this role than in an exploration of the true needs of their situation and of their patients. In emphasising the division between doctors and others, their training does not fit them to deal with patients, sickness or health.

There is a cost of belonging to this profession. The strength of the professional mystique means that physicians cannot afford to be totally honest with their patients or with themselves. The image of universal healer demands that he must have a solution for every problem. Clearly this is impossible. In practice it may mean 'a pill for every ill', some form of medical intervention when nature is adequate, or an increase in mystification[22] through psycho-analytical interpretation of symptoms. Should a physician admit that he cannot help most of his patients he sheds his protective mantle. This experience can be so shattering for the doctor that it leads to alcoholism or suicide. In Britain, suicide is more common among doctors than any other occupational group,[23] and the rate of alcoholism is exceeded only by that group of traditional drunkards, the journalists. One Birmingham general practitioner, whose suicide attempt failed, explained the problem:

> The general ethos of the medical profession . . . had led me to believe that in most situations the doctor usually knows best what is good for a person, and that because he knows best he is the natural head of the health team and his word is, or ought to be, authoritative.
>
> Trying to put into practice this 'cult of the expert' as a young GP led me into a lot of trouble and much personal distress. . . .
>
> My life gradually became one long psycho-therapeutic session from morning to night, occasionally interrupted by someone with a sore throat or appendicitis. I was, in fact, learning to play God and my patients were encouraging me to play the part.
>
> However, my constitution began to suffer, my blood pressure rose, my wife and child seemed to me to be more awkward every day and I began to use alcohol to try to escape from so many problems. Using/abusing alcohol caused me to have several road accidents which damaged other people and were very expensive. . . .
>
> The thought kept coming back to me that I know now also disturbs the minds of the most senior and caring men in my profession: that for all the work and all the deployment of my time and energy and expensive modern medicine, so little seemed to be achieved.
>
> The depressed women kept coming back for their antidepressants, the mentally handicapped children continued to have rotten educational opportunities. I seemed to have no effect at all on unhealthy ageing, accidents, heart and gut troubles.
>
> My total impotence in all this gradually became evident to me, so that after nearly ten years of dedication to the study and practice of medicine I came to the point of wondering whether I was of any value to anyone. The answer seemed to be 'NO'.[24]

When a doctor's reaction to the stress of his work is as extreme as this, his judgement is bound to be questionable. But even those general practitioners who are managing to cope may be dangerous if they cease to enjoy their work. Low job satisfaction is one possible result of the physician's failure to live up to his exalted image in Western society.

Dissatisfied doctors are particularly likely to prescribe drugs which have serious and well-known adverse effects, without making efforts to guard against the risks. High prescribing of practolol in the months before its withdrawal was associated with low job satisfaction. A similar pattern of dangerous prescribing has been found for a wide range of drugs. Dissatisfaction is also related to dubious aspects of practice management, including excessive use of ancillary staff to write prescriptions for hazardous drugs.[25]

Dissatisfied doctors may not end up by killing themselves, but while they practise medicine they may contribute to the death of their patients. General practitioners of a contrasting type have excessive confidence in their own judgement, they rely totally on their clinical experience and distrust 'book learning'. This faith in clinical judgement has been argued by the eminent medical sociologist Elliot Freidson to be fundamental to the maintenance of medical autonomy.[26]

Over-reliance on clinical experience is bound to lead to problems when dealing with rare events, particularly when the product life of pharmaceuticals shortens and at the same time more drugs become available. The opportunity to gain worthwhile experience fades against the commercial need for innovation. If this type of doctor dismisses warnings about drug dangers because he is overly swayed by his subjective beliefs about their value, his prescribing is likely to be dangerous.

Evidence of the hazards of over-reliance on experienced-based judgement comes from a study of the relinquishment of practolol in Britain. Doctors who believed most strongly in prescribing autonomy continued to prescribe practolol in spite of all the warnings they had been sent about its disastrous effects.[27] These same doctors were also more likely to prescribe barbiturate sleeping pills in the face of a long and widespread campaign against them.[28]

A selective memory among prescribers for the benefits of drug therapy as opposed to its risks can be predicted from psychological research. Added to this is the problem that people positively value the things they do simply because they do them. Just as heavy smokers will tend to avoid reading articles which tell them that cigarettes are dangerous, so prescription addicts fail to take note of warnings against over-prescribing.

Professional etiquette, autonomy and the sacrosanct nature of clinical judgement combine to allow dangerous prescribing practices to continue unchecked and uncriticised. The doctor is additionally protected by the confidential nature of medical practice. In most countries it is impossible to obtain a complete record of a doctor's prescribing behaviour unless he is willing to share this information. The more dubious his prescribing, the more defensive and secretive he is likely to be.

In Britain, some control over excessive prescribing is exercised by the Department of Health and Social Security, because it is this government department that eventually pays the drug bill for the National Health Service. Regional medical officers visit high prescribers to discuss their problems. Their effect is to reduce prescribing only temporarily. But the doctor's clinical judgement is sacrosanct, and doctors are not penalised for over-prescribing.

Despite its reluctance to criticise its members, the medical profession itself admits that over-prescribing is rife. Seeking a diagnosis for this malaise, some maintain that patients pressure them to prescribe when they would not otherwise do so. In fact, doctors prescribe more often than patients expect or wish, so some of the pressure does not come from the source to which it is attributed.[29]

It is nevertheless true that patients will consume more medicine than they need, and that there is a real patient demand for prescriptions. This is typified by the American patient who protested: 'Fifty dollars for a consultation, and all I get is aspirin? I want real medicine for that money.'

In the United States, Canada and Britain, around four out of five consultations in general practice end with prescriptions.[30] There are, however, enormous individual variations. One London doctor has become notorious among his fellows for prescribing for only one in five of his patients; others manage with little difficulty to achieve prescribing rates over 95 per cent.[31] These differences in overall rates attracted the detailed attention of research workers in the early 1960s but their causes remained elusive.[32] Differences in the make-up and morbidity of patient populations within an area were eliminated as being too slight to be significant, and the reason was traced back, not to differences in patients, but to differences between doctors.[33]

What is the seemingly compulsive mechanism that makes the prescription so predominant? Neither doctors nor patients are aware of many of the functions of the prescriptions they collude to produce.

Mickey Smith, Professor of Pharmacy at the University of Mississippi, differentiates between the *manifest* and *latent* functions of the prescription. Generally, only the obvious manifest functions are acknowledged; these derive from its documentary nature. They include its role as a means of communication about drug therapy, a legal document, a record source and so on. More important in producing problems of over-prescribing are the prescription's latent functions, of which he has identified twenty-seven. It is these that lead physicians and patients to use drugs when they are totally inappropriate for therapy. These functions are hidden but of nonetheless crucial importance.[34]

For the patient, one major latent function is the confirmation of illness. The prescription demonstrates to all that the visit to the surgery really was necessary. If the doctor refuses to prescribe, and offers no acceptable substitute such as hospital referral or tests, the patient would suspect that the reality or seriousness of the illness was not accepted. Without a prescription, the patient feels that he may have been seen as wasting the doctor's time. By giving the prescription the physician confirms that the visit was appropriate and that the patient may enjoy the status of what sociologist Talcott Parsons has called the 'sick role'.

Prescribing has clear advantages for doctors, and they cooperate with patients to produce this mutually desired outcome. It is a display of the doctor's power and privilege. Choosing drugs, writing and signing pre-scriptions, are beyond the capacity of lesser mortals. They are symbolic affirmations of the physician's professional position.

Control over prescribing represents the physician's capacity to control the consultation. If he offers only advice without a prescription, the doctor may feel he is lowering himself to the role of nurse or counsellor. In exchange for the acknowledgement of his position of power, and trust-worthiness, he gives a token, a symbol of his concern: the prescription.[35]

Increasingly, prescriptions take the place of any alternative forms of therapy, even when they are less appropriate for a diagnosis within the limitations of the medical model.[36] This is partly because it is easy to prescribe, it requires less thought and effort than a carefully explained suggestion about lifestyle change.[37]

Explanations are also less precisely defined in time: they can continue indefinitely without a clear end recognisable by both participants. Prescription-writing, by contrast, is ideally suited for marking the end of the consultation.

During the consultation, neither doctor nor patient may be aware of the significance of apparently minor actions. But through detailed study of videotaped consultations, sociologists have been able to analyse the inter-action between them.

Christian Heath belongs to a school of sociologists who use an ethno-methodological approach to interaction. This involves study of the minutiae of speech, gesture, and body movements to build up a picture of the way activities are carried out. A brief taste will illustrate this pains-taking technique; here Christian Heath is describing the way a physician gives a prescription to a patient:

> The practitioner rips the prescription from the pad. Concurrently the patient (having swung back in the chair) leans forwards, placing her hand upon the chair arm. The patient begins to lift her body and as she does, the practitioner thrusts the prescription forward in his right hand. As the practitioner thrusts forward, the patient's left arm and hand move to meet the practitioner's thrusting hand. At this moment the patient's standing is held, briefly, as she receives, in hand the pre-scription. Upon the patient's fingers closing on the prescription, both practitioner and patient retreat their hands. Immediately following the exchange and the practitioner's utterance 'right', the patient completes standing, turns away and leaves the room. The practitioner, uttering 'right', turns away, focusing gaze upon the patient's records. The terminal exchange occurs with the interactants turned away from each other.[38]

Heath comments: 'One finds that the very moves which bring the prescription-writing episode to a close are those that initiate the termination of the interaction.' He describes a ritual dance, where doctor and patient collaborate to produce a prescription, and to bring the consultation to an end after the prescription has been handed over.

Many physicians depend on using the prescription as a 'disengaging device' to shuffle patients through the surgery as quickly as they believe they must.[39] It has clear advantages, for the patient is not likely to know what effect the drug will have until it has been dispensed at the pharmacy, taken home and used. By this time the patient is out of sight and mind of the surgery.

From the consideration of the multiple role of the prescribing process it might be expected that individuals would develop their own prescribing habits, which would be followed with little regard for the symptoms presented by patients. Norma Raynes[40] studied general practitioners in London and found that massive differences in prescribing rates could not be explained in terms of the symptoms they were dealing with. There was also no relationship between psychiatric diagnosis and the prescribing of psychotropic drugs. Dr Raynes believes her data show that GPs develop particular routines which they operate regardless of the patients' presenting problems. Other research suggests that the proportion of cases for which psychotropic drugs are prescribed, which remain constant over time, is related to the doctor's own belief about the legitimacy of the use of such drugs,[41] and has nothing to do with the patient.

This is reminiscent of a classic study of physicians' judgements about the necessity for tonsillectomy for 1,000 school children. 'Of these,' the author reported, 'some 611 had had their tonsils removed. The remaining 389 were examined by other physicians, and 174 were selected for tonsillectomy. This left 215 children whose tonsils were apparently normal. Another group of doctors was put to work examining these 215 children, and 99 of them were adjudged in need of tonsillectomy. Still another group of doctors was then employed to examine the remaining children, and nearly one half were recommended for the operation.'[42]

These findings are problematic for those who believe in the reliability of clinical judgement and the importance of diagnosis. But they are consistent with research which has emphasised the importance of physicians' attitudes to their prescribing behaviour.

Repeat prescriptions for Valium and other similar minor tranquillisers are habitually used by some doctors in Britain to avoid seeing patients with demanding emotional problems. By allowing their ancillary staff to write prescriptions for such drugs, often for years on end, the doctor can avoid all contact with the patient.[43]

A group of general practitioners led by psychiatrist Michael Balint made a study of the repeat prescriptions they wrote. They found that the drugs prescribed were usually inappropriate to the patient's condition. The GPs saw themselves as struggling to treat frustrated patients for whom there was no satisfactory diagnosis, and hence no rational therapy. In these circumstances patients continue to attend surgery until a mutually satisfactory repeat prescription is negotiated. This takes the strain off their relationship, for the drug becomes a symbol of the 'something' the patient seeks. 'Peace is based on a precarious collusion . . . we think that in reality the repeat prescription is a diagnosis, not of the patient, nor of his doctor, but of the doctor-patient relationship.'[44]

If patients are vulnerable to repeat prescriptions, so may the doctor be. Acceptance of the blandishments of the pharmaceutical industry has been repeatedly shown to be associated, not only with poor prescribing practice, but with the use of dangerous and inappropriate drugs. Safer prescribers are more cynical about the drug industry, and are more likely to avoid contact with the detailmen.[45] One medical practice in Britain attempted an act of commercial sanitation, by completely isolating itself from all information from the industry. The doctors in this practice found that their prescribing rate dropped significantly.[46]

Other aspects of physicians' work situation are relevant to their use of dangerous drugs. Those who see more patients per hour prescribe to a higher proportion of them, they also do less thorough physical examinations.[47] Their patients inevitably return more often because there is less chance that the original trouble will have been identified. So these physicians set up a vicious circle, creating a heavier workload, which in turn leads to higher prescribing and increased risk because non-pharmacological options become more remote.

We have stated that the patient, or more correctly, the patient's condition, has little influence on the drugs he will be given; but he is not completely irrelevant. The physician's attitude towards different types of patient will measurably affect the sort of drugs they will be given. In one study it was found that GPs who preferred a pastoral role, acting as benevolent father figures, carried on prescribing methaqualone (Mandrax, Quaaludes) for much longer than colleagues who expressed more interest in internal medicine.[48]

Neither doctors nor patients operate in isolation. Cultural influences, the organisation of health systems and the economic background all affect prescribing.

Sometimes the variation need be very small to have a dramatic effect. Richard Dadja matched a group of doctors in England with a group in Wales on a minimum of eight out of ten characteristics, such as age, sex, nationality, size and area of practice and number of partners. He found that the English doctors prescribed 287 items for each 1,000 patients, whereas the figure for those in Wales was 590. He has not been able to explain this difference, but it is probably due to cultural differences between the two countries.[49]

Unfortunately the type of direct comparison Dadja was able to make cannot be generalised to other health delivery systems. For one thing, prescribing data are not readily available outside Britain. However, broad comparisons can be made. For example, West Germany is remarkable to students of prescribing for its medical profession's willingness to prescribe hypertensive drugs, that is, drugs to *raise* blood pressure.[50] In France doctors are twenty times more likely to prescribe vitamin B_{12} than their colleagues in the UK,[51] whilst the sensible Norwegian doctors prescribe antibiotics only half as often as their British counterparts.[52]

We can follow many strands of evidence about prescribing to reach the same conclusion. A drug is not the straightforward treatment for disease that it is usually supposed to be. The prescription is a product of the social interaction of doctor and patient within a particular culture.

Studies of the determinants of prescribing each provide pieces of evidence which go to form small coherent areas of the prescribing jigsaw. The complete picture of why physicians choose particular drugs for their patients will probably never be built up but a recognisable outline of the main features is already clear. Personality characteristics and social attitudes are the main determinants of what physicians prescribe. The patient's clinical condition is merely a contributory factor, one that is easy to overlook or ignore. Personal characteristics of the doctors have been found to be the only explanation for the variations in prescribing rates for particular drugs. The individual patient cannot play an important part. It hardly matters what the patient's symptoms are; the treatment offered depends upon the condition of the doctor.

Doctors are trained to fit into a professional role which effectively maintains their medical monopoly but which is not designed to benefit patients. Through years at an authoritarian medical school, idealistic young students are moulded into rigid doctors who have lost much of their original ability to empathise with patients and listen to their problems. Their determination is strengthened by a belief in clinical autonomy which allows then to apply an inadequate medical model in attempting to make sense of the problems that patients bring them.

So what is wrong, doctor? We suggest that the answer lies in the historical system that gains much of its strength from an inflexible approach to training, and infrequent reappraisals of the real problems confronting it. The medical student's social background makes him susceptible to this conditioning process. When the fledgling doctor emerges to confront the world of his patients, the very process of becoming a physician will have rendered him incapable of dealing with the majority of the problems that will face him. Because he is largely unaware of the forces acting upon him, the doctor has become, with the best will in the world, a significant force in the propagation of illness.

Nothing less than a revolution in attitudes will be required to correct the damage that is being done through over-reliance on drugs. Patients, society at large and the medical profession itself are being damaged. The corrective treatment could start with the profession. 'Physician, heal thyself.'

Chapter Eleven

People As Patients

Patients themselves cannot escape the charge that they, by their own attitudes and
actions, have contributed in a devastating fashion to the incidence of needless drug
use . . . They have pressured a physician to prescribe, even against his better
judgement . . . They have become prescription shoppers, going from one physician
to the next to obtain a multiplicity of medication.
— M. Silverman and P.R. Lee, *Pills, Profits and Politics*

The Western world has many myths about doctors, drugs and the efficacy
of medicine. Against this background, how realistic are beliefs about the
patient's part in the medical masque? The superficial view of the patient is
that through bad luck or unavoidable mischance, he has become ill, and in
being cured he is, for a short time, a patient. Reality is usually at variance
with this view. There are reasons for becoming ill; often the doctor is *not*
the most appropriate person to consult; and in very many cases not only is
a cure elusive but the consultation leads to a worsening condition and
perpetual patienthood.

The concept of illness requires clarification. Most illness is symptomatic: that is, it is in itself an indication of a deeper problem; but any
single symptom presented to a doctor must be treated at face value. A
clearly definable condition such as an infection or mechanical damage like
a broken leg needs little discussion; the treatment is obvious and straightforward. But if the doctor is consulted with one of a continuing series of
broken limbs or similar incidents by the same patient, it may be a
symptom of a social or psychological problem. Poly-symptomatic conditions are immediately more complex. Presented with a range of non-
specific symptoms, doctors base their treatment on a subjective assessment. Their treatment of such conditions – like 'anxiety', for which
millions are routinely medicated – must be largely idiosyncratic.

The particular symptoms suffered depend on as wide a range of factors
as the causes of illness. These include environment, lifestyle, culture,
conditioning and individual genetic predisposition.[1] Even fashion can play
a part; some of the symptoms commonly observed earlier this century
have virtually disappeared today, for example the total loss of sensation in
the hand and wrist once frequently associated with the unhappy state
diagnosed as 'hysteria'. On a shorter time-scale, the chain reaction of

illness in close groups such as schools, where one case of appendicitis is rapidly followed by many others, is well known. Equally well documented is the fashionable affliction, originally suffered by film stars or royalty, whose illnesses invariably stimulate a loyal outbreak of identical suffering among fans and followers.

Symptoms are very common in the general population. In a survey[2] concerned with health and medication, medical statistician Karen Dunnell found that 91 per cent of the population suffered at least one symptom of illness during the previous two weeks. She argues that at most, only one-third of these symptoms are taken to a medical agency, and that an individual's self-image is probably the most important variable in determining the reaction to symptoms. Those who see themselves as healthy consult doctors far less than those who do not, and the rate of consultation is not affected by the seriousness or frequency of symptoms.

To complicate matters further, symptoms themselves can show wide variation between individuals. This has been particularly apparent in studies of pain. Wounded soldiers in field hospitals have been found to complain of much less pain than civilians with similar surgical wounds.[3] This is thought to be related not to a tough military image but to the individual's perception of the meaning of the wound: the soldier was glad to be alive and safe whilst the civilian was ill and expected to suffer.

The concern of medicine with specific diseases and their symptoms and signs has obscured a crucial fact: people become clinically ill when they are subjected to any stress they cannot cope with. For example, a man whose wife has died faces a greatly increased risk of serious illness and death for the subsequent two years. The particular symptoms he experiences may seem to have nothing to do with his bereavement; he may develop cardiovascular or lung disease which could be attributed to years of smoking and breathing polluted air; he may fall victim to an infection which happens, at that time, to be epidemic; he may crash his car because of a lapse of concentration. We may live successfully with several factors which predispose us to disease, but an additional load can complete a fatal picture.

In the affluent world, the pressures leading to acute breakdown are primarily social and psychological. Particular social groups – the poor, the lonely and bereaved, oppressed minorities – are more susceptible. They have fewer ways of protecting themselves, fewer options are available, support systems are more fragmentary. These people are likely to find any life crisis harder to cope with effectively and they consequently experience more illness.[4]

This view of disease implies that symptoms are definite messages that should be heeded and interpreted. They are indicators that some part of the system is coming under an unacceptable load.

The problem may correct itself if symptoms are ignored. The body has enormous capacity for repair and regeneration. But unless the original causes of breakdown are eliminated or reduced below critical levels, illness is likely to recur.

For most of those who decide to consult their doctor, prescribed relief is purely symptomatic; it is designed to deal only with the symptoms offered by the patient. Medication may suppress symptoms but it will not affect their source, and the result can be indefinite drug use or the production of more symptoms as the body tries to reinforce its original message. A circle of increasing medication and proliferating symptoms is set up which can have no healthy outcome. Even treatment which is aimed at a perceived cause of illness – such as antibiotics for an infection – will not take account of the crucial precipitating factors which led the patient to fall ill. These may be themselves self-limiting; a long journey, sleepless nights and a foreign environment can conspire to reduce immunity to unfamiliar bacteria.

The pursuit of symptomatic relief solely through the use of medication is clearly unsatisfactory. Unless the condition is self-limiting, eradicating symptoms generally has one of two outcomes. Either the patient remains on medication in a more or less stable state of pharmacosis, or the condition worsens and the process of symptomatic relief is intensified. The best that can be hoped for is the permanent repression of symptoms at the price of becoming a permanent patient.

When the symptoms are seen as commonplace, acceptable aspects of daily life, the message they embody will be ignored. Thus the smoker will take no notice of a chronic cough, consulting only when he develops further symptoms. If he believes that his cough is an early sign of lung cancer which he imagines to be curable, he may not delay before consulting a doctor. If, however, he decides he has cancer and that there is nothing medicine can do to save him, he will not consult. And if he recognises that his cough is a warning that cancer may be the result of his foolhardiness if he fails to give up smoking, again he will not consult – unless he believes that a doctor can help break his cigarette addiction.

Consciously or otherwise, anyone who becomes aware of illness will weigh up the benefits and costs of following the possibility through by seeking medical or other help.[5] Among the potential benefits are the characteristics of the sick role.

Entry to the sick role is by way of consulting the doctor; the sick person is expected to try to get well by cooperating fully with medical personnel. In return, he is exempted from normal tasks such as going to work and relieved of responsibility for his condition and needs.[6]

To some, the dependent sick role is attractive in itself. Furthermore, patients have high expectations of the power of medicine to relieve discomfort. But these attractions are counterbalanced by widespread anxiety about seeing doctors. In a study of general practice, half the patients interviewed said they felt nervous about seeing the doctor: 22 per cent felt awe of doctors in general, 17 per cent were afraid of the outcome of the visit, and 12 per cent said the doctor's manner made them nervous.[7]

Many patients worry that their reason for consulting is not sufficiently serious to warrant the visit. Doctors are much more likely than patients to judge presented conditions as not serious, but they are poor at teaching their patients to discriminate between conditions for which consultation is appropriate and those for which it is not, even in a situation like the British National Health Service where there is no financial incentive for doctors to see their patients often. The general unwillingness of health professionals to share their knowledge is the single most common cause of complaint among patients.[8]

It is clearly impossible for the patient to force the doctor to divulge information, and awe will add to his difficulties. One patient's comment to an interviewer illustrates the problem: 'If you go to him he never tells you what you've got. I've never known him to say it was a certain thing. You always have to ask, and then he is very vague.' Another told how the doctor stalled: 'When I asked him about the tablets, about what would happen if I stopped taking them, the doctor only told me that I would become ill. I asked him in what way I would become ill and he said, "Oh, you will become very ill".'[9]

Whatever the communication difficulties, patients continue to approach doctors with trivial or inappropriate reasons. In Ann Cartwright's comprehensive study of general practitioners,[10] more than half the doctors considered at least 25 per cent of their consultations were over some trivial or unsuitable matter, and more than one quarter of the doctors believed that over 50 per cent were trivial. These opinions are associated with marked feelings of dissatisfaction on the part of the doctors. One GP said, 'I have to waste a lot of time on these people with a resultant loss of time for real patients and energy for study.' He thought that between 75 and 90 per cent of consultations were trivial, unnecessary or inappropriate. Among the trival consultations 53 per cent were minor illnesses which the doctor felt did not warrant medical care. These included colds, coughs, headaches, constipation and so on.

The doctor's problem is that his door is always open. For a lot of people it is the only door that *is* open to them. As our social structure produces more lonely and frustrated people, the traditional sources of comfort and assurance disappear. Families no longer provide the infra-structure of wisdom that was a feature of life a century ago. Today in urban society people are divided by age, income and status, and united by very little. Increasingly the doctor is asked to deal with problems that just would not arise with more tribal social structures.

Patients often mask the real reason for their visit with trivia. This is partly because they find it difficult to raise the problem, and they will offer the doctor a 'physical' symptom as something they can meet over, before admitting to the real reason for the consultation. It is 'dipping a toe in the water', a process in which the doctor's reaction is gauged and his likely reaction assessed. Stimson and Webb describe[11] how one patient began a consultation with a two-minute monologue on her menopausal symptoms. She then asked about her latest chest X-ray results, and finally raised the matter which particularly disturbed her, which was her daughter's illegitimate baby. Had the doctor seemed rejecting during her warm-up she could have cut off without seeming to be either foolish or to be wasting the doctor's time. An unknown proportion of apparently trivial consultations represent cases where the patient has felt unable to talk about the major problem which is troubling him.

With an open door, personal problems are often discussed with family doctors. Personal difficulties are undoubtedly important in the causal factors of disease, but the suitability of the general practitioner to deal with them effectively is open to doubt. Nevertheless he remains an available caring agency for many patients.

In these circumstances it is inevitable that social problems will take up a large amount of the general practitioner's time, unless his manner is hostile. If this is the case, the doctor can expect to find himself treating an unusually high proportion of apparently trivial ailments, each offered as an attempt to get past Square One.

A doctor who forces each patient into too small a consultation time-gap will constantly deal with 'false' symptoms, while the patient's real problem remains unresolved. Such doctors are likely to be high drug prescribers, because the medical problem offered as an opener may have an apparently suitable pharmacological remedy.

An illustration of this is the situation described by a general practitioner, Dr S. Gregory, in the affluent island community of Guernsey. He calls it 'the fat note syndrome':

> What about those patients who come back again and again with headaches, insomnia, abdominal pain, backache, constipation, vaginismus, palpitations and dizziness? The list is unending. All good physical stuff and all requiring serious attention – at first. Each new symptom warrants a full description and a battery of tests . . . The one or two abnormalities invariably found lead to more tests. The notes grow fatter and fatter.
>
> At the same time, or even in lieu of all this, comes treatment. Not knowing the diagnosis makes it difficult but seldom deters the doctor. The pressures are too great. 'Something must be done,' comes the

plaintive cry from those who have usually had too much done already.

The stage is set for the all too familiar merry-go-round. 'How did the pills work, Mrs Smith?' 'I think they helped my tummy, doctor, but now my feet are swelling'. Typical side effects; thank God her belly's better, thinks the doctor. At least I can get rid of the swelling with a diuretic and that will be something different to talk about.

And so it goes on, the tablet game . . .

In general practice I used to use the old ploy of handing them a bit of paper; more tests, pills, certificate, it didn't matter . . .

They would be back.

Dr Gregory is able to be honest about the syndrome because he has escaped from his complicity in the process. His patients benefited greatly from an hour during which they were allowed to talk freely about their difficulties. He comments: 'The funny thing is that they don't seem to come back, except for the occasional sore throat or broken bone.'[12]

Doctors are trained to treat patients, not to deal with people. When consulted, they tend to react by offering treatment whether the problem is medical or not. If the person finds the doctor's acknowledgement and attention in any way rewarding, then the cycle is likely to be repeated. The prescription is evidence of the doctor's concern, and the person will fulfil the role of patient to ensure that concern is forthcoming when required. 'Career doctor seeks career patient for lasting relationship, no previous experience or illness necessary.' They can go steady for a long time.

In accepting the small rewards of day-to-day involvement in the details of symptoms and treatment, both lose sight of the desirability of a real solution. For doctors, achieving professional status usually removes both the need and the capacity to question motives. As long as the doctor is in step with his fellows, following 'correct' procedures, he will receive their full support and be beyond criticism. Most seem quite happy with this situation and react negatively to colleagues who strive to solve patients' underlying problems or give them insight into the limits of the doctor's power. Dr David Ryde, a London general practitioner, whose approach is people- rather than illness-centred, prescribes at only 20 per cent of the national average rate although he has an average number of patients. Because he has fewer repeat consultations, he has enough free time to travel extensively and follow his other interests. He is deeply resented by his overworked colleagues.

It is easy to see how social routes to patienthood and sickness have developed. For the vast majority of consultations, the doctor is unable to be effective because medicine is not relevant, yet both he and his patient behave as if it were.

People become patients for reasons that are at best tenuously connected with the purpose of medicine; but drugs play an essential part in their conversion.

Social routes to sickness allow the worst abuses of the power of drugs. Drugs are used to avoid or 'solve' social or relationship problems, in the same way that doctors use them to 'cure' medical problems. The five modes below illustrate the operation of social conspiracies to turn people into patients. The complicity of physicians in these activities must be cause for concern.

Family, Mode 1   One member of the family unit makes it unstable: for example, the wife is unhappy and unfulfilled by her life within the marriage. Her expressions of distress are not acknowledged by the other members for what they are, because this would threaten the family unit in which they are quite happy. Instead they label her as 'sick', 'neurotic' or 'menopausal'. Uncertain that her complaints are justifiable, she gives in to family pressure and consults a doctor. He agrees that her behaviour is not 'normal', that she over-reacts, and he prescribes psychotropic drugs. These may sedate her sufficiently for her threatened withdrawal from her marriage/family role to be aborted. She will feel guilty about complaining, will be unable to deal with problems and will accept the sick role by giving up the fight.

An 'agony' letter from an angry husband and the published answer illustrate the early stages of one wife's likely route to illness:

> 'Can you please tell me how to get my wife to take more pride in her appearance and her home? About two years ago, I stopped her going out to work as she was neglecting the house and our two children. Our sex life is practically nil because she is always too tired. I help with the housework when I am not on night shift but she just doesn't seem to care, even to the point of not washing regularly.'

> 'In these circumstances there is only one answer: be completely outspoken. Suggest she sees the doctor about her tiredness and try to shock her into action by pointing out she will only have herself to blame if your marriage goes on the rocks.' (Katie Boyle in *TV Times*, quoted in 'Naked Ape', the *Guardian*, 26th October, 1981.)

Family, Mode 2   The marriage is under strain. Both parents concentrate their attention on the child, who is given contradictory instructions, and competing expectations, by each parent. The child is used in this way to bolster the ego of each parent. The child cannot cope and reacts by producing symptoms, like wetting the bed, that will remove attention from the marital problem by diverting the parents from their conflict. The child is put in the sick role to focus the anxiety of the parents, and the added stress that this puts on the child will increase symptom production. As an added bonus, rewards from parents for dependent, attention-seeking illness behaviour makes the sick role very attractive to the child.

Family, Mode 3   The children are getting bigger. Granny is no longer needed to baby-sit, and the eldest child needs more space. All the family feel the strain. The parents and children watch Granny closely for signs of 'no longer being able to cope'. Eventually Granny is driven into an old people's home, and if she had not used medication to bolster her through-out the battle, she will almost certainly succumb in the waiting atmosphere of the home.

Institutional, Mode 1: 'Nursing Homes'   Particularly a problem in the United States where age, like pregnancy, is treated as a sickness. Under Medicare and Medicaid old people qualify for higher funding if they are bedridden. They are also less trouble to the staff and cheaper to maintain. Chlorpromazine (e.g. Thorazine, Largactil) is the drug of choice because it is cheap, and it induces a state of sedation usually without putting the patient to sleep.

Dr Butler, Director of the National Institute on Aging, has described 'zombielike persons only dimly aware of the world around them' in United States nursing homes. 'You see people treated more for the advantage of the provider – namely, the administrators, the nurses, and physicians – than the patient. You can have a quieter atmosphere if you zonk people with medication.'[13]

Institutional, Mode 2: Prisons   In the USSR and Britain, difficult prisoners are given medication which incapacitates them. The medical profession is actively involved in this process. Prison Medical Officer Dr C.H. McCleery wrote: 'For some years we have had the problem of containment of psychopaths who, as a result of situational stress, have presented the discipline staff with control problems for which there has been no satis-factory solution. . . . *From a medical angle these men show no evidence of formal illness as such* [our emphasis] but, clearly, are characters having a lot of nervous tension, a certain amount of depression, considerable frus-tration with a low flash point who, until the situational stress can be removed or modified, are potentially either very dangerous or, in the case of the more inadequate, an unmitigated nuisance'. Dr McCleery added that those men 'are considered by governor and discipline staff as medical problems . . . and were regarded purely as discipline failures.'[14]

In this way prisoners identified as 'troublemakers', which must by definition include all prisoners, become 'medical' problems in need of treatment – known among British prisoners as the 'liquid cosh'. The doctors who allow it to be wielded must pose questions of acceptable morality at least as important as those asked of the drug industry earlier. If Valium controls the home and the street, Largactil is keeping the institutions quiet.

For those outside institutions who voluntarily adopt the role of patient, the benefits may include the social interactions with medical and ancillary staff for the lonely and unfulfilled, the drama and purpose of being a career patient and the well-known unlimited ability to discuss sickness and dying all the time. The unhappy middle-aged woman whose family is paying her less attention than she would like, and who is unable to substitute an alternative purpose in her life, is the archetype who adopts this career in the hope of satisfying her many psychological needs.

None of this is new. Many years ago, people would visit doctors and express vague dissatisfaction with life. The doctor would listen, diagnose something like 'nerves', and write a precription for some tonic, usually 'aqua pinka', or, if that did not work, 'aqua liq'. Pink or liquorice water was no more likely to solve the problems brought to doctors then than are the vast range of potent drugs now used for the same purpose. But it had one advantage: it was unlikely to cause any harm to the recipients.

Almost any encounter with a doctor will result in the offer of treatment. In a small percentage of cases this may be appropriate and helpful, but for the majority of people who consult doctors it will result in the pointless prescription of drugs. If this form of treatment is pursued without attempting to alter any of the factors that led to the need to seek a doctor's help, sooner or later the person will be turned into a permanent patient, suffering a perpetual series of illnesses.

Chapter Twelve

Consultations Like Clockwork

The physician who is an honour to his profession is one who has due regard to the seasons of the year and the diseases which they produce; to the states of wind peculiar to each country and the qualities of its waters; who marks carefully the localities of towns and of the surrounding country, whether they are low or high, hot or cold, wet or dry; who, moreover, takes note of the diet and regimen of the inhabitants, And in a word, of all the causes that may produce disorder in the animal economy.

Hippocrates

What happens after the patient closes the consulting room door behind him? Consultations are theoretically confidential, and often highly personal. Nevertheless, just as drug company detailmen have managed to get into hospital consultations, so an increasing number of sociologists, psychologists and doctors have penetrated the consulting room. Using sound and video recordings, they have been studying the detail of the interaction.

Patrick Byrne and Barrie Long became interested in this area through their involvement in training general practitioners. Their concern was to investigate the verbal behaviour of GPs in order to teach the next generation of doctors to be more effective. They comment in the foreword to their report that the doctor is 'Both a product and a prisoner of his medical education, which has made no attempt to provide him with behaviour suited to enable him to cope with psycho-social problems'.[1]

Seventy-one doctors from Britain, Holland and Ireland contributed tapes of their consultations for the study. The permission of all patients was asked, less than 5 per cent refused, and there is no evidence that either doctor or patient was inhibited by the presence of the recorder. Indeed the authors admit that 'the tapes contain consultations which may be described as professionally dreadful in terms of the skills or lack of skills shown by doctors . . . In a well-edited selection of tapes one would expect editors to try to eliminate their own failure at least to some extent.' As to the patients, they show a surprisingly wide range of behaviours, 'ranging from a lady wishing to know if the doctor would recommend a Hotpoint or a Tricity electric cooker to a series of the most harrowing interviews dealing with life-threatening situations'.[2]

Some consultations were categorised as 'completely dysfunctional'. The tapes reveal doctors failing to listen to patients, evading their questions, reinforcing their own position at the patient's expense and one characteristic of consultations that have broken down: doctor and patient talking at the same time, projecting their confusion onto the tape.

If doctors are to help their patients at all they must listen to them. Unfortunately they frequently fail to do this. The following example was taken from a consultation which Byrne and Long call 'otherwise quite normal':

DOCTOR: What time did the pain start?

PATIENT: I saw him at three or four in the afternoon . . . but he didn't seem to notice me then . . .

D: Yes, but what time did it start?

P: There was nothing to be said. Nothing at all [crying]. I wasn't there at first. It didn't seem real.

D: What?

P: When I came home.

D: At what time did it . . ?

P: It started at nine.

D: The pains started at nine?

P: What pains?[3]

Neither was listening to the other. The patient was very distressed, and the doctor was not pursuing what may have been crucial information. There are occasional consultations on record in which such non-communication goes on for two or three minutes.

This is an extreme form of a common type of consultation behaviour. More frequently the patient tries to raise a problem which the doctor does not wish to discuss; he will ignore it, fail to hear it, or persist with a different line of questioning despite the patient's offer. The following consultation comes from a doctor who is very much orientated towards organic concepts of illness:

DOCTOR: Good afternoon, and what is it you've come to see me about?

PATIENT: It's my eyes, actually.

D: Your eyes?

P: They are itching, smarting . . .

D: How long have they been doing that?

P: Oh . . . coming on for a week now . . . I don't know whether its worry, but Paul . . .

D: [interrupting] Have you been using any make-up?

P: No, I don't use make-up . . .

D: Because that is a very common . . .

P: No, I don't use make-up . . .

D: . . . cause of this sort of thing . . .[4]

The doctor persistently rejected the patient's offer of an emotional basis for her problem. The consultation ended with an unhappy woman leaving the surgery carrying a prescription which may or may not help the rash on her eyelids.

Some doctors show 'a remarkable inability to cope with anything but the most mechanical relationship with the patient'. Consider the following excerpt from a consultation involving a busy city doctor and a patient with many problems:

DOCTOR: And what are you on for your nerves?

PATIENT: I keep having very bad dreams every night since we've split up and I've brought these to show you what he's [another doctor, mentioned earlier in the consultation] been giving me, but I've still been having these bad dreams and I've been having these three times a day.

D: Do these seem to help?

P: Well, I don't really know. Well, obviously they must do.

D: Have you any children?

Later.

D: Well, I will give you something to sleep and something to calm you down and if these suit you we'll keep you on those but I think we'll change the . . . Do you feel it helps?

P: Yes, I do really. Obviously, I was very worried about this lump as well . . .

D: Mogadon?

P: Yes.

D: And instead of these Mogadon we'll just give you a capsule to take. This will help you to sleep. It isn't a sleeping capsule but it will help you to sleep, but it will also work during the day to try and lift this depression.[5]

Byrne and Long consider that at least 30 per cent of doctors would consider this consultation to be quite adequate, despite the fact that the doctor ignores the patient's desire to talk about a lump which has recently been removed from her breast. He also fails to follow up the bad dreams and the patient's transparent evasion of his question, 'Do these seem to help?'

Some doctors made statements of judgement about their patients which have clear relevance to the way in which they held their consultations: 'Treat patients like you treat drivers in front and behind – always expect them to do something stupid.'

'I see no reason at all to explain a patient's condition to him. If he asks an intelligent question I might offer some simple explanation – but on the whole I prefer not to.'

'How can you expect a layman to understand the sort of language we talk? Very few of my patients would have the faintest idea what was wrong with them even if I were to explain it to them.'[6]

The doctor who expected his patients to act stupidly, like other drivers, demonstrated a remarkable ability to see a patient every three minutes. Here is an example of his style:

DOCTOR: Good morning. What is it then?

PATIENT: I've got some sort of inflammation here. I'm not sure what caused it but it's not too comfortable.

D: Yes. Let's have a look. Mmm. Mmm.

P: Do you think it could be caused by those tablets I started last week?

D: No. Turn round. Let's have a look at the back of the leg. Mmm. Mmm.

P: Well, it all started twenty-four hours after I changed tablets.

D: Those tablets have no side-effects.

P: What's side-effects?

D: Never mind. Can you walk comfortably?

P: Yes, I can't wear those heavy winter underpants though. Do you think it's caused by wool or something like that?

D: No.

P: I got soaked last week, I fell into a gutter and had to walk home all dripping wet. Is that it?

D: Maybe. Right. Take this to Mr . . . [the chemist]. Rub it on until it's gone.[7]

This astonishing consultation demonstrates the doctor's willingness to be unhelpful, rigid and dishonest – the latter when he stated that the tablets had no side-effects. His only concern was to hustle the patient through the consultation.

Time pressure is the explanation usually given by doctors, and often accepted by patients, as the reason for inadequate investigation of the patient's complaint. It is likely to be partly responsible for the known relationship between high prescribing rates and short consultation times. Short-consultation doctors are also more likely to feel dissatisfied with their work, to cut corners and to feel burdened by a high proportion of trivial complaints.[8]

For some doctors management of time becomes of paramount importance. Effective operation as a doctor is characterised by a 'quick clean job'. A doctor who sees an average of fourteen patients per hour believes: 'A doctor's primary task is to manage his time. If he allows patients to rabbit on [talk continuously] about their conditions then the doctor will lose control of time and will spend all his time sitting in a surgery listening to irrelevant rubbish.'[9]

A consistent characteristic of the many dysfunctional consultations quoted is that they finish with a prescription which may be used in an ill-judged attempt to resolve the conflict by dismissing the patient, even if his problem has not been dealt with. Such prescriptions are unlikely to satisfy the patient, who will most likely return for a further consultation, perhaps to see a different doctor. A patient interviewed in a study by Fitton and Acheson expressed her resentment at being fobbed off in this way:

'He didn't tell me anything. Just gave me the prescription. He's writing out the prescription as he's talking to you. He just doesn't seem to listen.'[10]

Questions about drug side-effects or about more serious adverse reactions very rarely arise in general practice. In every case noted by Byrne and Long where such issues do come up, the topic is quickly dropped. Only *one* doctor was even prepared to accept the possibility:

PATIENT: I'm not too keen on tablets.

DOCTOR: No, and quite right too. We eat far too many tablets you know. *These are quite safe I only prescribe these now you know.* You'll see, you'll sleep like a top.[11]

Dr Mulroy, a Yorkshire GP, made an attempt to study the effects of the discovery of iatrogenesis in his practice. He found that 2.6 per cent of his consultations were the result of iatrogenic disease. These cases put considerable pressure on the doctor-patient relationship, which is generally not of the quality that can tolerate any additional strain. He found patient reactions varying from aggression and suspicion to further regression into illness. For his part the doctor 'usually felt guilt and this manifested itself as either anger, usually towards the patient, or over-activity in care'.[12]

Inevitably the strain on the doctor-patient relationship affected subsequent consultations. The recurrence of iatrogenic disease in the same patient brought the doctor to regard such patients as 'awkward' or 'neurotic'.

Dr Mulroy quotes the case of a young woman who, he considers, exemplifies the problem which arises through iatrogenic disease:

A 23-year-old married woman was an 'ideal' patient. Shortly after becoming pregnant she developed acute cystitis which was treated with sulphamethizole. Seven days later she developed a generalised irritating maculopapular eruption (skin inflammation). She was reassured, the drug was stopped, and she was given promethazine hydrochloride (an antihistamine) to relieve the irritation. Within ten to twelve days she felt quite well, the eruption subsided, and she went sunbathing. Within a few hours she developed an acute photosensitization which resulted in some blistering of her face, arms and feet. This may have been due to either the promethazine or the sulphamethizole. Four months later on in the pregnancy she was noted to have iron-deficiency anaemia. She was given intramuscular iron (iron dextran) and developed an acutely tender nodule in the right buttock. She was concerned at the possibility of developing a sarcoma (a tumour) in that site. Her confinement proceeded normally. When the child was four months old he developed an acute respiratory tract infection which responded well to ampicillin. Within four days treatment had to be discontinued because of severe diarrhoea and obvious candidiasis (thrush) of the mouth and buttocks.

Her requests for visits are now usually late and there have been several calls 'off the street'. Consultations are conducted in an atmosphere of suspicion, mistrust, and a mild degree of aggression on the patient's side and hesitation from the doctor's side.[13]

Despite Dr Mulroy's heightened awareness of the problem of adverse drug effects, his relationships with patients who suffer from them became difficult. His awareness leads him to comment: 'Throughout the duration of this survey one gained the impression that a patient who had suffered one iatrogenic episode was more likely to suffer another.' He did not seek to measure recurrent rates, but other studies seem to indicate that some patients are more likely to suffer adverse effects than others. In a small number of cases, patients will produce an adverse reaction to almost any medicine, a reaction akin to the cure achieved by placebos.[14] In practices with less enlightened doctors such patients inevitably come to be regarded as nuisances. Too often the label 'neurotic' is substituted by doctors for diagnosis and understanding, especially when the doctor believes that the drugs he prescribes are totally safe, or that he has never seen an adverse drug reaction.

From the patient's point of view the doctor's response to symptoms of drug-induced disease can be shocking. The prescription of tranquillizers may be underwritten by the inference that the patient is irrational or mentally unstable. Or the doctor may simply refuse to treat the patient, telling him to go elsewhere with his problems.

Even before problems of iatrogenic disease arise, many physicians are on the defensive. Rather than work with their patients and keep information flowing both ways, they will use predominantly doctor-centred behaviour. The goals of this behaviour are as much to fit the patient into the doctor's priorities, whether efficient time management or the promotion of cold baths, as to produce genuine improvement in the patient's condition. If we still believe that the point of the face-to-face consultation is to achieve effective health care, then it must be acknowledged that the style and techniques of most doctors have the opposite effect. And the ending of a dysfunctional consultation with an inappropriate prescription compounds the likelihood of iatrogenic disease for the patient.

Feedback from patients about the effects of medication is often treated dismissively by doctors. Inevitably this will reduce the detection of drug-induced disease, and it will also tend to make patients more anxious about offering important information to the doctor in the future. One young person quoted by Fitton and Acheson said: 'They're in a position of authority. They have power over you and know everything about medicine. I don't know anything.'[15]

When patients do find themselves driven to challenge the doctor or to demand that he discuss a question that is important to them, they may be faced with a sharp rebuttal: 'I am the doctor and I will do whatever prescribing needs to be done.'[16] One doctor said to his patient: 'I will tell you what is wrong with you, I will tell you what your symptoms are and I will tell you what to do. I am the doctor here and you will kindly not forget that fact.'[17]

The stories told by iatrogenesis victims in Chapter Eight now take on overtones of sad familiarity. To suggest to a doctor that his treatment has caused illness may constitute an unacceptable challenge. But when treatment for your illness has made you sick, and your doctor rejects you, to whom then can you turn?

Chapter Thirteen

To Whom Can We Turn?

Most victims of drug-induced disease turn to nobody for help, usually because the cause of the illness is not recognised. Few doctors and even fewer patients will accept medicines as the cause of their ill health. And if the question is raised perhaps by a relative or parent, as with Joan Daniels, who asked if her baby's congenital abnormalities were caused by the drug she took during pregnancy, the answer is only likely to reveal ignorance of the subject coupled with a denial of the possibility.

The majority suffer the conditions they develop without question. If they are elderly it simply becomes part of an accelerating progress towards death. If they are young, corrective surgery or rehabilitative support may be possible. But most drug-induced diseases are so insidious in character that doubt about their cause will always be present. This means that for the greater proportion of iatrogenic disease, whether recognised as such or not, the doctor will be the first person the symptoms are taken to, and he will prescribe more medicines to alleviate them.

A patient suffering from diuretic-induced diabetes would be treated in the same way as any other patient suffering the same disease, whatever its cause. The treatment of diabetes, as with most illness, is symptomatic. The cause is generally unknown and considered irrelevant. The bias towards treating symptoms and ignoring causes is characteristic of Western medicine, and this bias is maintained in the treatment of disease caused by previous treatment. Thus the circle becomes progressively more vicious for the patient.

If a doctor accepts the possibility that his prescribed treatment may cause adverse reactions among some of his patients, is there anything he can do to prevent this? With some drugs adverse reactions are so common that a process of therapeutic anticipation has developed between the discerning physician and the drug manufacturers. This provides a generally satisfactory answer for both of them, usually in the form of joint therapy with two or more drugs. The first will be given for the original complaint, and the second to treat the anticipated reaction to the first. Sometimes both drugs will be given in one tablet. A simple example is Navidrex K, manufactured by Ciba, a diuretic with potassium contained in a slow-release wax core. As potassium is lost from the body due to an unwanted side-effect of the diuretic, it is replaced by the core of the tablet.

This may appear a simple way to solve a problem, yet the fact that such drugs can pass the regulatory requirements means that adverse reactions are accepted as part of everyday drug therapy; and this acceptance allows some manufacturers to take particular advantage of some of the unwanted properties of their products. Squibb produce a modified tetracycline called Mysteclin, which includes the fungicide nystatin. This is designed to eliminate the yeast super-infections which occur when the bacteria which normally control them have been killed by the tetracycline.

Any particular drug is rarely vital to a patient. When an adverse reaction occurs, the obvious remedy would be to remove the cause of the problem by taking the patient off the drug. But unrecognised addiction can cause new problems, as graphically recorded by Barbara Gordon in her book, *I'm Dancing as Fast as I Can*. Ms Gordon started taking Valium for a back problem. Over ten years, the dose was slowly increased as she found that larger and larger quantities were necessary to ward off panic attacks – symptoms from which she had not suffered when she began to take the drug. Eventually she came to believe that she was dependent on a drug which was no longer an answer to her problems. On confronting her doctor with this realisation she was told, 'They are not addictive. They can't hurt you.' Her interpretation was rejected; she was classed as 'hysterical' and offered stronger medication. Finally she made up her mind to stop taking Valium. Because of her addiction, the result was total breakdown and serious psychiatric problems lasting several years.

Despite this risk with some types of drug therapy, there are signs that the radical approach of therapeutic withdrawal is gaining credibility. For some patients in residential care, withdrawal from as many drugs as possible is the first step in a curative regime. Psychiatrist Dr James Folsom, who directs ICD Rehabilitation Center in New York, has pioneered drug-free treatment for the elderly and for mentally disturbed patients of all ages. After entering his Reality Orientation programme confused and sick on polydrug 'therapy', they can be returned to rational functioning by being treated as human beings.[1]

If a patient suspects that new symptoms are the result of drug therapy he is likely to confront his doctor with this suspicion. The doctor may reject the proposition, or change the drug, hoping this will solve the problem. More probably he will react with some degree of rejection of the patient. This rejection may settle into the 'truce', based on unlimited and inappropriate repeat prescriptions, described by Balint's group.[2] One victim of drug damage felt she was 'being treated like a leper', and this may be an accurate comparison. The doctor keeps his distance, and gives whatever the patient needs to go away. In much the same way medieval monasteries had a lepers' gate, where food and water in non-returnable containers would be pushed to sufferers across a closed 'cordon sanitaire'. This sort of arrangement allows both monks and doctors to fulfil their obligations with the minimum of fuss and contact.

In extreme cases the doctor will totally reject the patient. This may be done directly, the physician advising or instructing the patient to go elsewhere, because he can 'do no more' to help, as with Mrs James in Chapter 8. Or the doctor may behave in a way that drives the patient to go elsewhere. Either way it is obviously a traumatic experience for the patient to be rejected by the very person he trusts will help to heal him at the time he is probably really ill.

In the United States, the question of trust has been shown to be crucial, for it is when trust breaks down that patients are likely to initiate malpractice litigation. Generally, patients are willing to accept failures in medical treatment as long as trust is maintained. Doctors who are prone to malpractice suits are those who are unable to maintain empathy in their relationships with patients. Both litigation and failure to pay medical bills have been linked with dissatisfaction resulting from the breakdown of communication between doctor and patient.[3]

Can causing iatrogenic disease, and then ignoring or improperly treating it, be considered grounds for a complaint of malpractice? The first, and usually insurmountable, difficulty faced by the victim of iatrogenic illness who wishes to take action against a doctor is to get confirmation of the cause of his condition from another doctor.

Should a patient consider he has a complaint against his physician, he will usually find machinery exists to allow it to be pursued. It is part of the structure of a professional body to provide for complaints against its members. At worst this is good public relations and at best it allows the traditional 'bad apple' to be removed from the otherwise wholesome barrel. But when a patient decides to use this machinery to seek redress he will find himself facing a system totally loaded against him. Under a veneer of reasonableness, every step will be designed to put the patient off. In his book 'Complaints Against Doctors',[4] Professor Rudolf Klein describes the British system in detail. The complexity of the process is frighteningly obvious from the diagram opposite.

The experience of a Plymouth family illustrates some of the problems

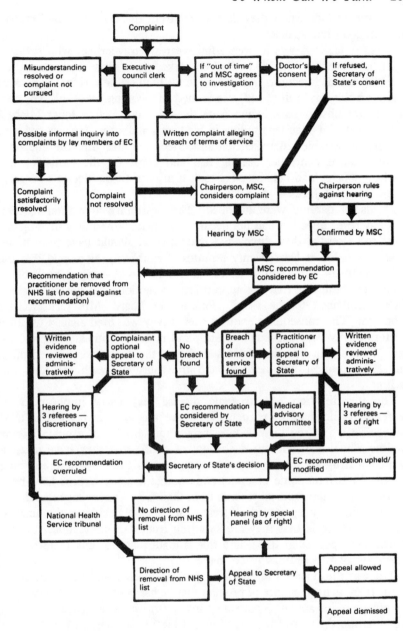

Diagram 10. The British Complaints Procedure. After Klein, Ref. 4.
MSC – Medical Services Committee, a sub-committee of the Family Practitioner
Committee.

that patients face when they dare to confront the medical establishment after tragedy has struck.

Michael Jackson was a twenty-four-year-old trawlerman who suffered from hay fever, for which he had embarked on a series of desensitizing SDV (Bencard) injections. According to his mother, he was 'in the peak of health on this day, full of fun, sun-tanned and looking beautiful'. His own doctor was absent so a locum gave the injection. Before long, Michael complained of a peculiar tingling in his hands and arms. He was given an antihistamine tablet. Between ten and fifteen minutes after the injection, an ambulance controller, eating fish and chips by the roadside, saw Michael stagger and collapse. He took him back to the doctor's surgery, where Michael Jackson died.

Michael's parents were horrified. The possibility of a fatal reaction to a hay fever injection had not occurred to them. When they investigated their son's death, they discovered that Michael should have been under observation for at least twenty minutes after the injection, and that the only treatment for a reaction was adrenaline, with oxygen available if necessary. Believing that the appropriate precautions had not been taken, they complained to the Family Practitioner Board. Mrs Jackson later reported: 'The consequent enquiry was heavily weighted against us. Five doctors to my very nervous husband, and no other witnesses allowed for us.' Without the ambulanceman's evidence, the doctor was cleared of all fault. An inquest was refused, and the cause of death recorded was asthma.

The identification of iatrogenic disease may carry implications of professional negligence, particularly where the drug involved was used unnecessarily, in too high a dose, or for too long.[5] Unfortunately some victims who know without a shadow of doubt that they have taken a particular drug are unable to prove it when it is denied by the prescribing doctor. In Britain some practolol and vaccine damage victims have been unable to get their medical records from their GPs. Others have found that doctors failed to keep records of treatment. The only evidence that may be incontrovertible is that they are suffering from damage identical to that caused by a particular drug, and this is inadequate for any realistic consideration of proceedings to be made.

If it was the doctor's intention to provide 'proper and necessary treatment' there is little chance of proving that he has been negligent, whatever the effects of his action. A statement in the British Parliament summed up the situation thus: 'Neither the National Health Service (on behalf of the doctors) nor anyone else can insist on medical infallibility, and a failure to reach the right conclusion cannot as such be held to be a failure of the doctor's obligation under the NHS.'[6] Clearly complaints about inappropriate therapy are likely to fail.

It is universally true that, provided the doctor sticks to the rules which define his function and behaviour fairly closely, the open-ended possibilities of his actions are not his responsibility. There are variations in different countries, but the doctor's position is underpinned by the acceptance of his right to 'clinical judgement'. All professional bodies have their self-protective codes. The doctor's position is unique, however, because of his powers of life and death.

In theory British victims of drug treatment are as free as any others to sue their doctors for negligence. However their chances of success may be less than in other countries. For one thing, British law, in common with many other legal systems, does not require a doctor to be correct in his judgements. In Britain, as in the United States, the test for medical negligence is whether the doctor acted in accordance with accepted medical practice. In a recent case, Lord Justice Lawton pronounced that an obstetrician's decision, which led to the birth of a brain-damaged baby, 'was based on his clinical judgement. Neither he nor any other doctor can always be right. Being wrong is not the same as being negligent.'[7] To win a malpractice suit in Britain is therefore almost impossible. All the physician needs to do is to argue that he treated the patient to the best of his ability and that, in his clinical judgement, the treatment was appropriate. The outcome of the treatment is immaterial.

Unless a doctor has broken the law or the ethical standards of his profession, and can be proved to have done so, his position is pretty watertight. But one possible chink in his armour has not been explored, and that is in the area of the authority he delegates to his ancillary staff. It is a common practice for doctors to issue repeat prescriptions, or to permit ancillary staff to issue prescriptions on their behalf to long-term patients on regular drug therapy. The situation has arisen where a regulatory statement is made about a drug, and the doctor is duly informed, but the doctor has not informed his ancilliaries who continue to prescribe the drug without special supervision after its hazards are known. Does this constitute a sufficient basis for action against the doctor? It has yet to be tested in the courts.

Many of the problems faced by patients in Britain are shared by those in other countries. It is an ideology common to both medicine and law which operates against them. The United States offers most hope for victims; the law generally is more equitable and also more accessible. It is possible to initiate a medical malpractice suit on the basis of damage caused by inappropriate drug therapy. By its nature private medical practice is not amenable to the same monolithic controls and protections as socialised medicine. Under a free enterprise system the doctor or his insurance company is much more exposed, whereas with state medicine the attack on a doctor tends to be deflected towards his employer. Under either system, doctors are allowed to sidestep the attack, which is borne by their insurance company or professional association.

Whatever the system of medicine, the government is inevitably involved. In the United States this interest devolves upon the individual States, who both operate welfare provisions and control the system of licensing for physicians to ensure that only those with appropriate training and qualifications are permitted to practise. Generally the licence is issued by the State in which the physician chooses to practise, although States do have reciprocal agreements which allow them to recognise other States' licensing. A complaint against a doctor can lead to the revocation of this licence, and other penalties. Naturally each State has its own complaints procedure.

In New York State the Health Department handles complaints against doctors. It may act if a patient brings to its attention any of a range of illegal practices. These vary from practising with 'incompetence' or 'negligence', or refusing to provide medical services to a person because of race, colour, creed or national origin, to 'unethical' conduct, such as revealing information about a patient without permission.

Under this system problems with drug treatment may be deemed to have resulted from incompetence or negligence. Complaints are handled first by an investigator, who, by acting also as an arbitrator, may be able to resolve the problem with the doctor. If the complaint stands, it is reviewed by a Screening Committee, which may request further information from the parties involved. If the Committee decide the complaint has merit, the Health Department's Counsel will prepare charges against the doctor, and the case will be presented on behalf of the Attorney General. It will be heard by a Hearing Committee with a totally different membership to the Screening Committee. In this procedure the complainant becomes a witness, and is not expected to battle against the profession. The Hearing Committee will make recommendations on the case to the Commissioner for Health, and submits a report to the Board of Regents who make the final decision on guilt and penalties. This is an involved and time-consuming procedure, and its effects, as far as the patient is concerned, may be intangible.

For understandable if rarely valid reasons, patients do not wish to blame their physicians. To lose trust in the healer is much more dangerous to the individual than to blame a business corporation. Hence action for legal redress is far more often threatened, or taken, against drug manufacturers than against doctors. The frequency of such actions is a reflection of the legal system of the country in which the lawsuits are brought. They are most common in America, where lawyers will accept cases on a no-fee basis if they believe there is a chance of winning a share of the damages. Thus relatively poor people can sue large drug manufacturers with a hope of success. British law, as we have seen in the case of practolol, requires that the patient prove that the company was negligent. To avoid this it is only necessary for a manufacturer to take reasonable care.

The concept of 'reasonable care' is obviously a matter of opinion and open to a variety of definitions. And the skill of the Counsel engaged would obviously be of tremendous importance in the outcome of any case which hinged on such a phrase. Skilled barristers are expensive, far beyond the means of all but the most exceptional drug victim, yet well within the grasp of the drug industry. The system of financing legal action in Britain militates against its use. The cost of a case is unrelated to its outcome, and British solicitors generally work on a cash basis. A lawsuit against a drug manufacturer is not a realistic proposition for a drug-damaged person in Britain.

However there are exceptions, and these expose a further defensive mechanism of the manufacturers. This is illustrated by the litigation in the High Court between Mrs S.L. Lawley and E.R. Squibb & Sons Ltd, concerning Squibb's antidiarrhoeal Quixalin (halquinol) and its alleged effects on Mrs Lawley's eyes. Litigation ended in February 1981 after terms of settlement had been agreed by both parties. The terms of the settlement included a mutual undertaking on confidentiality, although the company has not admitted liability nor accepted that Mrs Lawley's injuries were caused by Quixalin.[8] Obviously a settlement under these conditions can effectively prevent any discussion of the dangers that may be involved in the use of a particular drug.

This rare case is particularly interesting, in that it led to an even rarer event. Dr Hansson of Göteborg, Sweden, and Dr Herxheimer of London, had been asked to appear as expert witnesses for Mrs Lawley. They took the unusual step of publishing what amounted to their evidence in the *Lancet*. The authors claimed that 'settled cases are usually buried in silence, even when they are of far-reaching importance, as in this case'.[9]

Having thus effectively broken the silence, they revealed that it was claimed that Squibb had failed to take account of the toxic qualities of the closely related drug, clioquinol, and reference was made to reports from the 1960s showing that halquinol had produced blindness in calves, and severe hind-leg paralysis and sensory disturbances in dogs. Squibb's 1965 submission to the then voluntary Committee on Safety of Drugs for a product licence for halquinol mentioned toxicity studies in calves, but apparently not that they went blind, and was not explicit on the paralysis found in dogs. The authors add: 'Other documents showed that in 1971 Squibb was seriously considering the implications of the Japanese SMON epidemic and had drafted a warning paragraph for inclusion in the package insert. However, that warning was not included until more than six years later, in March 1977.'

Immediately after the settlement of Mrs Lawley's case it was discovered that another British case of optic atrophy associated with halquinol treatment had been known to Squibb since 1975, and was listed in the CSM's Adverse Reactions Register. The reporting physician provided the court with full details of the patient, and correspondence with Squibb discussing the case. It was considered 'disturbing' that Squibb did not disclose this to the court. Halquinol is no longer marketed in Britain, though it is still said by Squibb to be manufactured in Britain for export, mainly to South America.[10]

Even the thalidomide tragedy did not lead to a lawsuit against Distillers, the British manufacturer. But increasingly, victims of adverse drug reactions are overcoming the inherent bias of the British legal system by seeking to sue companies in America when the parent company is there. A current case has been initiated by British victims of oral contraceptives. They have employed a New York law firm to act for them against the American head office of the British subsidiary who supplied the Pill. In this way they hope to exploit the greater freedom of American legal processes, and also to use the different information and warnings issued about the product in both countries, as significant evidence against the drug manufacturer.

In most European countries legal action against drug manufacturers is equally difficult. In Germany the first thalidomide case dragged on for years, never reaching a final settlement because the plaintiffs were unable to continue indefinitely. The company finally offered to settle out of court with the victims and their representatives. This pattern was repeated in other countries including Sweden and Britain.[11]

Settlement out of court is more common than conclusive litigation. It has many advantages for the drug companies. It is likely, on balance, to be less expensive than a long-drawn-out trial, and it has positive public relations potential. The company can point to its generosity in giving compensation for injury to a drug victim without the compulsion of having been proved legally liable. However, such donations are made entirely on the company's terms, they are generally conditional, and may be offered or refused in an arbitrary manner. Moreover they fragment the opposition to the company, and once more cast drug victims into the role of supplicants. Thus out of court settlements can actually strengthen the interests of the pharmaceutical industry, while defusing the protests of their victims and the complaints about their products.

Within the EEC proposals have been made which would create a more equitable system, at least in theory, for the individual. These involve the application of the principle of strict product liability. This would mean that the manufacturer would be liable if any patient suffered an adverse or unpredicted side-effect from a drug. The full proposal includes the right to compensation for all victims.[12] Predictably campaigns have been mounted against these proposals by both the medical profession and the drug manufacturers. The benefits of a system of strict liability for Europeans are unlikely to be realised in the foreseeable future.

In Sweden the government has established a scheme that is almost comprehensive. To finance this, drug companies pay a proportion of their sales income, equal to about 0.8 per cent, into an insurance scheme. This 'voluntary drug product liability scheme' started in July 1978. It is designed to cover all serious drug injuries, including those suffered during participation in clinical trials, and victims may have the assistance of the State Patient Ombudsman with their claim. In the scheme's first twenty months it handled 215 claims,[13] against a background of 2,409 reported adverse drug reactions in Sweden during 1979.

Any compensation scheme must cope with the problem of identification, as many adverse drug reactions are indistinguishable from other illness. When some drugs marginally raise the statistical probability of contracting a particular common illness, it is impossible to say whether a drug was the cause in an individual case. The Swedish scheme demands that the cause-effect relationship between drug and injury be established. Of the 158 claimants whose adverse reactions occurred after the scheme began, seventy-three were found to have injuries that did not warrant compensation because the level of effect was judged to be 'acceptable', too short-lived, or the connection with the drug was dubious. Clearly the scheme allows for considerable discretion in its awards, and like compensation schemes set up by drug manufacturers, an unknown number of victims will be left without compensation.

It is a feature of voluntary schemes that they are perceived as unjust. If there is the slightest doubt about causation, the inherent bias acts against the patient's interest. In Britain, the thalidomide 'Y list' of deformed children to whom Distillers refused to pay compensation became notorious because their undeniable injuries highlighted the arbitrary nature of the scheme.

Even when they get the maximum amount of compensation possible, many victims do not feel satisfied. Perhaps this is because they are denied the dimension of vengeance. Their injuries are permanent; the company's losses are transient.

For the victim, getting money from a voluntary scheme involves reliance on third parties. ICI will not consider a practolol claim unless the victim first provides a letter and completed form from his GP. Naturally, many of the physicians involved refuse to provide such evidence, nor, in Britain and in many other countries, is there any way of compelling them to do so. They apparently fear that it will be taken as an admission of guilt, and may be used against them in some unspecified way. But without this cooperation even a victim of the unique and unmistakable oculomuco-cutaneous syndrome, with the full pattern of eye and ear damage, and internal sclerosis, will not be considered.

Whatever the outward appearance, getting compensation will involve a fight. And it will place stress upon drug victims which they may be in no condition to cope with. At what may be the lowest time of their lives they will be expected to move into totally unfamiliar area of knowledge and experience. Success will demand perseverance and fortitude that may be more appropriate to saints than to demoralised and perhaps frightened drug victims. It is little wonder that many stoically suffer in silence.

One answer to fighting against overwhelming odds alone has been for the victims of particular drugs to band together. Whilst singly they may not possess the necessary strength, morale or money, as a mutually supportive group with an understanding of each other's circumstances, they do. In their search for strength they find each other.

To some victims, emerging from isolation by such contact, the knowledge that others understand and care is enough to change their lives. Joining together enables them to pool resources and information, and share the burden of seeking legal aid. A group is also much more likely to attract the interest of the media, and once their story begins to be publicised by the press or broadcasting it attracts other victims, and positive action becomes a possibility. Fifty people have more credibility than one, and a hundred are on the way to being a movement.

As iatrogenic disease has grown, so has the number of victims' groups. They tend to be informal *ad hoc* organisations, concerned only with the issue of their particular injuries from a particular drug. In South Wales, practolol victims have organised themselves into a group which holds regular meetings. These are organised jointly with the solicitors negotiating compensation claims and the local Community Health Council, and occupy themselves with progress reports on claims and the exchange of information on medical specialists. They also provide a forum for social reassurance and contact.

Their group interests do not extend outside the questions of compensation and the effects of practolol, but national groups are springing into existence to deal with the problem on a wider scale. The Eraldin Action Group in Britain was coordinated by Jean Trainor, who became involved because her mother suffered serious eye damage from the drug. For some years all Jean's spare time was spent in correspondence and on the phone, organising and communicating from the front room of their small terraced house in a suburb of Birmingham. With minimal resources she performed many vital functions for practolol victims, one of her most crucial roles being to act as a friend and counsellor for many hundreds of victims who felt dismayed and isolated by their injuries. When they told their stories to her, she did not react with the disbelief they so often faced, but with practical help, advice and contacts.

Similar action or interest groups have been formed around other drugs. For example, by parents of vaccine-damaged children, who have been able in some cases to get compensation from governments, where vaccination was a part of health policy. Parents of children who were damaged when their mothers used hormone pregnancy tests have formed an association to further their childrens' interests, as have women who have been damaged by the contraceptive pill. Specific drugs, such as the long-term contraceptive Depoprovera, are also attracting groups who are opposed to their use. The numbers of action, interest and opposition groups grows as drug use, and drug damage, increases.

Although these groups may ease the burden upon a victim by support and contact, they cannot undo the damage that the drug has done. The groups that exist are brought into being by very serious drug problems for which there is little hope of reversal or cure. The victims, like Mary Wilkins whose case we have already discussed, can perhaps make their biggest contribution by informing others of their plight, and making the dangers of iatrogenesis known as widely as possible. It is a course which requires considerable courage. For themselves the best that drug victims can hope for is a little money to make life easier.

People addicted to drugs are in a different position. Although not usually physically damaged, they are none the less prescription drug victims, and some groups or self-help organisations are able to offer real support and hope of a cure. Victims are usually addicted to minor tranquillizers which are not immediately hazardous. For that very reason they have been prescribed so casually that quite a different type of problem has finally been recognised: pill dependence. Barbiturate sleeping pills are well known to be addictive, and the risks involved in withdrawal from them widely documented. More recently, the ubiquitous everyday benzodiazepine tranquillizers and sedatives, Valium, Librium, Tranxene, Dalmane, Mogadon and so on, have been admitted to be the drugs of addiction of probably 3 million Americans.[14]

Regular use of benzodiazepine tranquillizers is similar in effect to regular alcohol use. For some addicts the two are interchangeable, and heavy, but costly, drinking is used to bridge the gaps between prescriptions. Pill and alcohol cross-addiction is now common. When violence, blackouts, erratic behaviour and slurred speech make the existence of the problem undeniable the only answer may be detoxification in hospital. This is as unlikely to provide a long-term answer for the pill addict as it is for the alcoholic.

Some of these drug victims have joined groups like Pills Anonymous, which, like its forerunner Alcoholics Anonymous, involves regular meetings of addicts and ex-addicts. The members are respectable citizens whose problems began with a prescription given to them by their well-meaning doctor for anxiety or associated symptoms. Probably the pills helped them to bear the anxiety, and then became the crutch on which they came to depend. The first prescription was followed by repeats, with the quantity of drugs used growing as habituation and tolerance grow.

Pills Anonymous (PA) offers a route to a pill-free life, by substituting a religious crutch and a measure of self-reliance.[15] PA is growing in America, and alongside it Pill-Anon, a support group of family, friends and concerned people, which again parallels the work for alcoholics' families of Al-Anon. Some bodies formed for other problems are redirecting their concern to prescription drug victims. An example is the Heroin Addiction Unit in New York where staff have been transferred to work with tranquillizer addicts. Perhaps this is more than usually appropriate, since the Medical Director of Roche Pharmaceuticals is a member of the advisory committee. Ex-addicts are forming groups to help themselves, like First Step in London, set up by two young women who had been dependent on a range of psychotropic drugs. Yet whatever the outcome of the work of these groups with individuals, it is unlikely that they can have any influence on the original cause of drug dependence. Ultimately the graffiti advice in the drug-aware 1960s still holds true: 'Do not adjust your mind, reality is at fault'.

The development of interest groups concerned with specific drugs is paralleled by the growth of consumerism in medicine. The battles of consumer groups usually occur on the periphery of the medical industry, and are predominantly directed towards reinforcing regulatory and control functions; making sure the rules are observed and people kept on their toes. Consumer groups tend to have no ultimate aim and therefore are locked into a dependent position of permanent opposition.

Nevertheless medical consumer power has had some impact on drug manufacturers. Ralph Nader is synonymous with outspoken consumerism, and in the United States his Washington-based Public Citizen Health Research Group, headed by Dr Sidney Wolfe, campaigns on all aspects of health care. Part of this work involves gathering information about drugs, and using it to force the Bureau of Drugs to act on safety problems.

The Health Research Group has been active since November 1971. Since that time its director and his associates have demanded controls over the use of drugs ranging from Alka-Seltzer to sex hormones. The FDA has been presented with evidence of imminent hazards, and demands for total bans on the prescribing of chloroform, clofibrate, Darvon, Flagyl, Ilosone and oral anti-diabetic drugs. In the face of inaction, the Health Research Group has sued the FDA, a step it took in March 1976 over chloroform, which is believed to cause cancer. A lawsuit was also initiated against the

University of Chicago and Eli Lilly on behalf of women given DES in a 1950–52 experiment.

In Britain consumerism is undeveloped, and aggressive consumerism practically non-existent. The Consumers' Association does produce the Drugs and Therapeutics Bulletin, but its influence is restricted. Its style and content are aimed at doctors; in fact the government Department of Health and Social Security buys most copies to distribute to doctors.

The development of positive consumer activity depends upon access to information, and in this, Britain is different from the United States. Government in Britain is characterised by secrecy. America, by contrast, has a Freedom of Information Act, which allows anyone, even a foreigner, access to administrative records and the people involved. The FDA is open to approach by the public on any matter; the CSM is not. It does not communicate with the public; indeed it is difficult to find out on a casual basis who is in charge of the various functions it performs. Fundamentally the difference is a reflection of the fact that Americans are citizens, with rights, whereas Britons are subjects, with duties.

At a more political level organisations such as New York's Health Policy Advisory Centre (Health/PAC) and Britain's radical Politics of Health Group reflect concern about medicine in general. For such groups the issues are the political philosophy controlling delivery of health care, and the economic influences on the propagation of both health and illness tend to be important. Obviously in this context medication is just one aspect of the larger problem of a medical system which is perceived as misguided. While drug victims may use the perspectives developed by such organisations as these to understand the basis of their current problem, they will not find much practical help.

Whatever their virtues, consumer groups cannot be of much direct help to the drug-damaged individual. They look for improvements in control and regulation to minimise dangers, ensure better public protection and bring about changes in emphasis. Where they are concerned with pharmaceuticals they also seek a reduction of the power of the pharmaceutical industry, and a concomitant increase in the power and position of the consumer. They are not necessarily concerned with the basic problems of drug use. Essentially the message of medical consumerism is 'more, but better, please'.

Consumer, patient and victim groups fight discrete battles against various manifestations of the megalithic drug industry. Each tends to be engaged in a limited skirmish with a system that is built on excessive drug use. Those who concentrate on the evils of long-term Valium use would not suggest that drug treatment of high blood pressure, or upper respiratory tract infections, is often equally irrational and hazardous. They rarely challenge the underlying rationality of the Western approach to medical intervention.

No group has become sufficiently detached from its immediate circumstances to offer a serious challenge to the drug-dependent system as a whole. Each reacts to the part which has injured its members, while encouraging those parts which have not. The magic bullet has penetrated deeply. We encourage the search for anti-viral agents, for anti-cancer drugs, without questioning the factors that make the drugs appear necessary in the first place. We welcome the pill that will make life easy, a chemical tint, if not a bed, of roses, despite the damage that the last one did. The fundamental truth is ignored. Effort and resources are squandered on disjointed repair work inspired by the wisdom of limited hindsight. Patching over faults is usually necessary when the fabric is unsuitable or rotten.

In the final analysis is there anyone a drug victim can turn to? Each potential helper is limited by his assumptions and the constraints of his position. The physician by his training and limited perception, the legal system by its preoccupation with money, fellow victims by their own survival problems and a lack of clarity about where blame for their situation lies. For many victims there are feelings of guilt. The original purpose of their visit to the doctor that began their progress down the iatrogenic trail may not have been necessary at all.

But how many people who become patients realise all that is involved? Injuries, insidious and continuous ill-health, premature morbidity and death, questions of politics, multinational business and medical ethics – these are the principal strands in the tangled web which begins to be woven for every patient who takes prescribed drugs inappropriate to his condition.

Others may be there to shoulder the blame for our misplaced trust. But in the end we must turn to ourselves.

Part Four

Possibilities and Perspectives

Chapter Fourteen

Possibilities and Perspectives

It may appear that the message of this book is absolutely anti-drug. This is far from the truth. Our attitude may be stated thus: that properly tested drugs, correctly applied under skilled supervision, can benefit humanity. We would argue with the drug industry, the medical establishment and the consumer, on questions of emphasis and scale.

We believe that what is required is a major change in fundamental attitudes to medicine and medication. If the usefulness of drug therapy is not to be obscured by the excesses of its application, a drastically altered perspective of its potential is needed. To achieve this the whole Western concept of medication must be considered in the broadest possible way. Procedural or regulatory adjustment or onerous restrictions on usage are not in themselves the answers. A radical reappraisal of the place of drugs in industry, in medicine and in life in general is required.

Growing disquiet is being expressed about the problem of drugs. Usually this is voiced as a plea that their application be tempered with realism and rationality, but criticism at this level ignores the nature of the forces that lock drug use into its present pattern. The manufacturer seeks the maximum profit for his product, the doctor uses this product because of its inherent power and convenience, and the patient takes it in pursuit of a cure or an altered social role.

The overall problem with drugs has arisen because each group is concerned exclusively with its own particular interest, and has been content to take on trust the involvement and integrity of the others. The only exception to this are some regulatory agencies, which have tended to become repositories for the conflict created by the dichotomy of interests felt by governments.

These conflicts have limited public debate on drugs to questions of their price. Even these debates are narrow affairs, seldom questioning basic discrepancies such as international price variations. Generally it is considered that drug prices are too high, and manufacturers are accused of making 'excessive' profits. Yet surely the achievement of the best price and maximum profit is an essential part of the Western world's free market economy? Is it fair to criticise drug manufacturers because they play the game too well? If these criticisms are valid the only option would seem to be to accept the exceptional nature of the drug industry, and control prices on some entirely arbitrary basis. This degree of rejection of the capitalist philosophy inevitably produces unsatisfactory compromise. The British mechanism of VPRS has produced a *de facto* partnership between government and industry, to the benefit of the latter with negligible effect on the drug bill. The Swedish compensation scheme, which taxes manufacturers on their drug sales revenue to provide funds for victims, simply passes the cost of damage on to the consumer. State control of the drug industry is a consideration beyond the scope of this book, and we offer no opinion on its desirability.

Problems posed by the use of therapeutics force us to consider one key issue. It is that the 'free enterprise' commercial corporation may simply be the wrong kind of social institution to produce useful medicine. There are too many built-in contradictions and basically opposing concepts. Profits, monetary efficiency and competition do not generally equate with care, compassion and healing. To expect a profit-motivated organisation to work for individual welfare may be as unrealistic as expecting the average alligator to be a good babysitter. It is just not the right sort of animal.

For individuals, the crucial issue is better health. It must be accepted that very few modern pharmaceuticals have anything to do with promoting health. They are predominately concerned with servicing illness by masking symptoms and creating illusions. Cures are rare, but cushions and crutches abound in the pharmaceutical armoury. The question must be answered: are drugs now doing more harm than good?

If health is to be improved by the consumption of drugs, new criteria must be accepted for their use. The first and most urgent is that of *absolute minimal medication*. Minimal use of medication will require a conceptual shift by all the interests involved, and may therefore be considered hopelessly idealistic. Nevertheless we believe it is the only sensible philosophy to adopt. Practically we could begin by accepting that a substance may only be used therapeutically *if it has proved benefits*. This seemingly obvious requirement goes far beyond what is demanded of any drug today. In Norway the authorities demand that there should be a therapeutic *need* for a drug, but the proof of the fulfilment of that need must be doubtful because of the multiplicity of factors hindering accurate assessment, not least the unsatisfactory nature of clinical trials. In America the FDA stops short at *efficacy*, that is, the drug must do what the manufacturer claims it will. This does not involve the concept of benefit, only that of honesty, and again proof rests with the unsatisfactory clinical trial procedure.

On a world scale it would seem rational if existing agencies such as the WHO were to be strengthened and given a regulatory role which was accepted by governments, including those who benefit financially from the export activities of their multinational corporations.

Poor countries need protection from the excesses of the drug industry, and carefully controlled exposure to drug therapy. In the industrial countries reliance on drug therapy followed *after* the major public health measures had been taken; in the third world the reverse is true. When the WHO states that 80 per cent of the disease in the world is attributable to the lack of a clean water supply, the application of drugs is like building on quicksand. Governments must be encouraged to rise above the corporate desire for profits to ensure that benefit results from the activities of their industries.

It has been estimated[1] that in America and Britain the majority of physicians prescribe a range of only forty to fifty drugs. For countries requiring a basic yet comprehensive pharmacopoeia, the WHO provides a list of 250 drugs, five times the number regularly used by the average physician. In view of this does the availability of more than 25,000 therapeutic substances make any sort of sense? Rational application of essential drug therapy is being hindered by the enormous amount of litter on the pharmaceutical landscape.

Our assessment of the use of drugs has led us to the conclusion that, with benefit, prescribing could be rationalised at around 20 per cent of its present level. The British drug bill of £1,000 million could be reduced to £200 million. The problem is that the only group whose interests would benefit from such a course of action is the patients, and at present they have very little say in the matter.

Rationalisation of use does not always reduce costs, and some consumers may have to accept that although the potential savings on a national scale are vast, the price of some drugs could increase dramatically. Properly used, many drugs would cease to be an attractive commercial proposition, because the quantities needed would be so small. This could lead in turn to the renaissance of the small effective specialist manufacturer, who would not create the problems generated by megalithic multinational corporations.

When criticised, drug companies frequently defend themselves by reference to their dynamic research and development functions. But close examination indicates that the majority of products evolved in company laboratories are principally concerned with ensuring the health of the company. Fundamental research into areas of genuine medical need is both costly and high risk in nature. At present the majority of this type of research is not undertaken by the drug companies but by university departments, to which the industry may make donations, but from which the results are made available at no charge to the industry. It has been argued that most of the significant pharmaceutical innovations of the past thirty years have been discovered in academic institutions, and then exploited commercially by the drug companies.[2]

If this is the case, would it not make sense to rationalise the situation by removing research and development functions in medicine from commercial corporations? Research could then be carried out by genuinely independent academic bodies, guided by established medical need. The benefits of patents derived from such research would produce income for the research body which would enable it to become self-financing and thus protect necessary high risk projects from direct commercial considerations and grant dependency.

Drug manufacturers would then simply be drug manufacturers. Companies could bid to produce drugs at the lowest sales price to the consumer, while guaranteeing a royalty income to the patent holder. Manufacturers would then concentrate on those areas of expertise required to produce and distribute, efficiently and cheaply, drugs for which there was an established need, and therefore minimum financial risk. Their profitability would depend upon their competitiveness as manufacturers.

This scheme assumes the desirability of a national context for the drug industry. Currently it is dominated by multinational giants who benefit from their ability to manipulate the universal desire for their products. The advantages of the international need for medicine could be decisively realigned by arranging intranational manufacture through a body such as the WHO, allowing it to receive a percentage of the royalty income due to the patent holder by acting as an honest broker. It would be able to channel medical needs from parts of the world without research and development capacity to those with such abilities. Thus the skills and medical expertise of the developed countries would be used for the mutual advantage of both rich and poor, and the 'drug colonialism' and arrant exploitation of the underprivileged would be reduced considerably.

Similarly the burden of damage caused by drugs, which at present is left firmly upon the victim, would be more susceptible to redress. It is clearly inequitable that obtaining compensation or assistance for people so injured should be so extremely difficult. Attempts to adjust the balance of advantage in favour of the consumer inevitably founder on the present corporate structure of the industry and the organisation of the medical profession. The rationalisation and devolution described above would assist by allowing clear areas of responsibility to be defined.

The research and development organisation would be responsible for complying with the standards defined by the government regulatory body to achieve a licence to market the product. The manufacturer would be responsible for adhering to the standards, formulae and procedures specified by the licensor, and any additional requirements that the regulatory authority may demand.

Finally the regulatory body, which has licensed the drug and agreed to the conditions for its use, must accept responsibility for any damage caused by the drug, provided the doctor has prescribed it correctly and the patient adhered to the therapeutic regime. With this responsibility the regulatory body would need teeth and facilities to safeguard itself, and in so doing it would protect the public who rely upon it.

When a drug disaster does occur in spite of all safeguards – and this will always remain a real possibility as long as new medicines are used – the government of the country or countries concerned must accept responsibility. It is the government which benefits via taxes from the commercial activity involved, and it is also the government which is responsible for the activities of the regulatory body which has licensed and monitored the product. Throughout the nineteenth and twentieth centuries governments have progressively taken more responsibility for the health of their citizens or subjects. It is illogical for them not to accept responsibility when health provisions fail individuals.

The solution of the drug problem will require major conceptual shifts. Such shifts will be hindered by the enormous and incredibly powerful forces which have created the problem, and wish to maintain the *status quo*. These include the medical establishment, the pharmaceutical industry, and governments. And it cannot be denied that large numbers of people, who may or may not be patients, have tremendous faith in the present medical care system, and they add their weight to its inertia.

Nevertheless we believe firmly that the drug industry emerges as a liability. Not only to health and adequate medical care, but to the community's financial welfare. The continuing increase in spending on medicines involves paying more and more to achieve less and less, a classic situation of diminishing returns, which ignores the basic requirements of treating illness and promoting health.

A realistic perspective for a typical drug may be this: correctly applied to 2,000 people it could be a lifesaver; given to 2 million it could do little harm, if little additional good; but when it is produced, promoted and irrationally prescribed for 20 million it is almost certain that it will do more harm than good.

In the short term any rationalisation of use requires the rationalisation of information. Most countries do not know how much of how many drugs are being consumed, and have no way of knowing what effects the drugs are having on their populations. Use is based purely on an *assumption* of good. At present it is difficult for anyone except trained specialists with access to appropriate data to make any judgement on widespread drug effects. Even in sophisticated countries the information is far from complete. America has to rely on market surveys to guess how much of each drug is used. In Britain prescribing data are available in the form of a comprehensive computer print-out, 'List D', but the information is protected by the Official Secrets Act, which is supposed to be concerned with inhibiting acts of espionage. Only the manufacturers know precisely how much of each drug is produced and marketed.

In the face of the multinational nature of the drug industry, some tentative moves are being made by national regulatory bodies towards co-operation. These are directed towards information sharing and the achievement of common criteria for accepting new drugs onto the various national markets. Predictably little progress is made. From a meeting of thirty-three national regulatory bodies sponsored jointly by the FDA and the WHO and held in Maryland from 28th to 31st October 1980, the most positive thing to emerge was agreement to publish a list of all the participants.[3] Cooperation founders because the priorities of the regulatory bodies are distorted by the needs of their parent governments, and these are frequently at variance with both the best interests of their populations and the international common good. In this regard the British government is notably one of the most culpable. Its love of secrecy has led it to avoid making information available to the FDA because the US Freedom of Information Act would make it accessible to the public.

The British lack of openness operates to favour the interests of the pharmaceutical industry over those of patients throughout the world. If a companies applies to the CSM for a product licence for a new drug and the CSM refuses it, the company can withdraw its application. Officially, no decision is taken under these circumstances. This procedure allows the company to deny that the application has been rejected in Britain when it seeks to register the drug in countries which specifically ask about the outcome of applications to other regulatory bodies.[4]

A similar mechanism operates when established drugs prove to be dangerous. Manufacturers can quietly withdraw them without informing anyone of the real reasons. The CSM has been criticised by the WHO and the EEC's Committee for Proprietary Medicinal Products (CPMP) for failing to report the withdrawal of products from the British market. Should the CSM take regulatory decisions of this nature, it is required by international agreement to inform the WHO and the CPMP so that other regulatory bodies are warned of the potential hazard. Voluntary withdrawal avoids this disclosure.[5]

Concerted international action on hazardous drugs is further hampered by the confusion engendered by the multiplicity of names used for each drug. Although a drug will generally have only one generic name, it may have many different brand names in each country, giving the possibility of hundreds of names for the same substance all over the world. In Britain aspirin appears under 104 different trade names. In addition, active drug ingredients may be included in many different combinations, each spawning a further multiplicity of names in each country. Thus even when a clear decision is made about a drug, tracking down all the possible sources of the danger is far from straightforward.

Yet it *could* be a simple job. The computer is the ideal tool for the data handling and reviewing task involved. At present computers are used to build 'drug profiles' by regulatory agencies, and some attempt is made at coordinating the results of this work by the WHO. However its potential value is not realised because its scope is too limited. Whereas drugs are available on a world scale, monitoring and information processing remains a parochially national affair. Hence Norway has a particular computer system for the drugs and information considered relevant to that country, and the United States has a different system for handling what is in essence the same information about the same drugs. This diversity creates an obstacle to the free flow of information.

If information is to reach all users, a common generic name should take precedence over the manufacturer's brand name in all labelling, listing and prescribing. The only convincing argument for brand names is a commercial one. This logical continuation of computer listing into everyday usage would enable every consumer to know exactly which drug has been prescribed, discussed or warned against. Such an extension of knowledge and debate into the public domain would require a considerable change in attitude by doctors, the pharmaceutical industry and all those concerned with medicine. At present the consumer is regarded as a passive, almost incidental, part of the medication process.

For the doctor the obvious problem posed by the pharmacological avalanche is in information handling. Drug innovation and renovation together with patients' histories present a picture of ever increasing complexity. Doctors protest that they just do not have instantly available information on adverse reactions, side-effects, interactions and contra-indications. While computers are under-used as electronic filing systems in a growing number of practices, they have only recently been used to manipulate the sort of information the doctor should ideally have at his finger tips.

In Britain, Dr Bob Johnson, a general practitioner, has developed a desk top system which is programmed to take patient records, therapeutic and drug history, current therapy, symptoms and other information which is then instantly available to the doctor.[6] Any change in the patient's condition or therapeutic regime is fed into the system, which will automatically warn of potential problems such as possible drug interactions or contra-indications to proposed therapy. The programme base includes current drug data which is constantly updated, and which could be linked directly to a central drug information system.

If this system were generally available the doctor's surgery computer terminal would become the input point for monitoring all aspects of drug usage, allowing the rapid building and review of the performance profile of any drug. Even a subtle effect, like the increase in death-rate from all causes found in the WHO clofibrate study, would be detected by such a system. Conversely, any unexpected and unlooked-for benefits of a particular drug would be picked up as deviations and brought to light for development and further evaluation.

Only a system of this sophistication will give reliable data on the risks and benefits of drugs in general use. The data base of the national regulatory agency would be able to draw on relevant experience of every patient in the country. And from the national base the international co-ordinating body would have access to information about the effects of drugs used by patients in all countries with computer technology. Although the initial cost may seem high, we believe such a system would rapidly pay for itself by the more rational use of drugs, and a reduction in the expensive after-care required by those tens of thousands of people currently damaged by drugs. There appears to be no other practical means of tackling a problem with the dimensions presented by drug abuse. If banks and other financial institutions can profitably use equivalent technology on a similar scale, surely we can afford to do so in the cause of decreasing illness?

The introduction of computers into medicine, as with other areas of human activity, is viewed with suspicion. But there can be no denying the advantages of a direct link between the prescribing doctor and the latest information on the drug he proposes to use, and his ability to match its action to his patient's susceptibilities and requirements. Dr Bob Johnson has made what he calls the 'pen and pump' analogy. In London in 1849 an epidemic of cholera fever was stopped by Dr John Snow who intuitively recognised the water from the Broad Street pump as its source. By removing the handle from the pump, Snow stopped the spread of the disease. Dr Johnson believes iatrogenic disease will not decline until the pen is removed from the hand of the physician, forcing him to accept the logic, discipline and advantages of computer technology.

Any analysis of the misuse of drugs must find fault with doctors. As controllers of the prescription pad they choose to overuse drugs. Instead of acting as a protective filter between the drug industry and their patients, doctors have opened wide the floodgates. They have allowed themselves to be persuaded, cajoled, pressured and educated into taking the apparently simple course of prescribing drugs whenever they are faced with a patient.

But the doctor is struggling with an impossible job. He uses tools which are unsuitable and concepts which are no longer valid, and consequently fails as a healer and a promoter of health. His profession relies on a simplistic view of man which distorts the human animal into subdivisions of anatomy, biochemistry and physiology. Social sciences and psychology are acknowledged but usually dismissed, and medicine is dominated by clinical experience and judgement tempered with science.

This approach to medicine is founded in Cartesian dualism, the philosophical system developed by Frenchman René Descartes (1596–1650). The recent upsurge of interest in 'holistic' solutions to problems is the first sign of displacement of his system. Cartesianism presented two parallel but independent worlds, of the mind and the body, each of which could be studied without reference to the other. Accordingly the mind does not directly move the body, nor the body affect the mind, although both may react together. The second characteristic of Cartesianism is a rigid determinism, in which living organisms are governed by the laws of physics and there is no need of a soul to explain the actions of animals. Descartes made a slight exception to this rule for man, whose soul he believed resided in the pineal gland of the brain. His followers soon discarded this inconvenient anomaly in the system.[7] Both the germ theory and the magic bullet fitted perfectly into this philosophical structure. Chemotherapy seemed to be rational and scientific.

In his ascendancy the doctor has inherited many of the functions previously filled by the parish priest. He looked after the bodily, emotional and spiritual health of his flock, seeing them as interrelated. But a mechanic for the human machine is patently unfitted for coping with a broad pastoral role. The doctor frequently feels he cannot solve the problems that are brought to him. What can he really do for death, poverty, unemployment, unsatisfactory housing or fundamental problems such as over-population and starvation? On an individual level when confronted with the fear of disablement, ageing and death all he can do is blunt the perception to reduce the pain. The struggle to behave as a scientist working within the Cartesian model has resulted in frustrations for the doctor and iatrogenesis for the patient.

Doctors need to be re-educated about drugs and their place in therapy. It is assumed by most general practitioners that their use of drugs is, by and large, rational, even 'scientific'. In our discussion of the variability between doctors in prescribing habits and the factors which determine it, we showed that this is very far from the case.

This is a fundamental message which must be understood by doctors, otherwise they limit their discussion of drugs to narrow issues, like the choice of the 'best' antibiotic to treat a specific infection. Such questions, like those about the price of drugs, distract from the major issues – is a drug necessary, will it do more harm than good, is it appropriate to the patient's problem or merely to his symptoms?

Doctors must raise their sights from the servicing of illness towards the promotion of health. As a first step they should remove themselves from involvement with trivia and routine. Chronic illness may demand constant medical attention, but there is no reason why this should involve the doctor. Usually his skills are not needed, while the patients' needs remain unsatisfied. In these situations nursing and trained ancillary staff are more appropriately deployed, so long as they have ready access to a doctor if necessary. Such staff are able to advise the diabetic, assist the arthritic and check on the hypertensive. Doctors must recognise and resist the temptation to take over large areas of minor responsibility.

Similarly the pharmacist, with highly specialised skills and detailed knowledge of drugs, could be given much more control over medication. Professor Mickey Smith has pointed out that the pharmacist is often the only person who can keep track of all the various drugs taken by most patients, and that to use pharmacists simply to distribute drugs is 'a tremendous social waste of trained manpower'.[8] He offers a range of possible models for more appropriate use of the pharmacist's skills, proposing that the pharmacist could be totally responsible for drug therapy following a physician's diagnosis; or that he should, at least, have a quality-control role, monitoring drug therapy but without personal responsibility for choice of therapy. A health care team approach where the patient benefits from the combined expertise of doctor and pharmacist would be ideal.

For while doctors may maintain a degree of medical monopoly, they should not have a health monopoly. Their role must change and become more educative. In between the surgery and the hospital there is an obvious need for a real health centre, with facilities for active teaching about health and related matters, such as diet, exercise and environment. It should include a gymnasium open to everyone, but where special attention can be paid to the needs of identifiable groups such as hypertensives, people with cardiovascular problems, pregnant women and others for whom defined types of activity are essential.

As fitness and regular exercise are fundamental to health, so are emotional well-being and social integration. Community or tribal lifestyles hold many lost keys to man's health and happiness. Many people whose problems could be alleviated or solved by social contact find it difficult to break through barriers created by their condition. Frequently the basic problem is isolation, so a health centre must avoid the hierarchical institutional approach which either repels, or further isolates them within its self-perpetuating mechanisms.

Physical health cannot be separated from all the other aspects of the human condition. The practice of medicine will only be effective if its perspective is changed from crisis intervention to the long-term promotion of health. In such development the role of the physician would remain crucial. His education and insight would make him the key figure in a network of caring and health promotional staff. A multiple-function health centre, based in community or neighbourhood, would provide enhanced opportunity for the practical application of doctors' skills, whilst allowing capacity for overview to develop away from the trivia that presently clutter their working lives.

Many problems currently taken to general practitioners could be helped by counselling. Emotional, sexual, marital and family problems may require the availability of trained counsellors for their solution. Doctors, as we have seen, are usually not suitable people to deal with personal problems. If counsellors and medical staff shared premises, in relaxed informal surroundings, not only would appropriate problems be more likely to be brought for counselling, but the doctor would be able to pass clients to the counsellor, and vice versa.

General practitioners will protest, as they do when confronted with any proposition requiring change, that they do not have time, or resources. Treating their patients is a total preoccupation requiring all their energy. This has been shown to be a misconception. Nevertheless doctors often feel threatened by the thought of sharing knowledge. Their monopoly of knowledge maintains the awe in which patients hold them, and mystique is fundamental to their professional status. The derivation of the title 'doctor' incorporates the ideal to which Western medicine must return; doctor comes from the Latin *docere*, to teach. The doctor must become the prime motivator in encouraging patients to learn to maintain their own bodies and minds.

One English medical practice has discovered the advantage of teaching patients about minor illnesses. Geoffrey Marsh, a GP in the relatively poor and high-morbidity area of Stockton-on-Tees, described the strategy:[9]

After a brief history, patients who appeared to be suffering from minor self-limiting illness were carefully examined. Increasingly the examination was preceded by comments such as 'from what you tell me I don't think I'll find anything', so that with a similar history subsequently patients would feel that consultation would be unnecessary.

Convincing reassurance was then given about the minor importance of the illness, including a detailed account of its expected course. The rarity of the forty-eight hour 'flu was emphasised, and patients were taught that some minor illnesses may drag on for two or even three weeks. Indications for re-consultations were spelt out. The value of medicines in treating such illnesses were discussed, and most were dismissed as possibly offering some slight symptomatic relief but as often with some unpleasant side-effects. The place of common-sense home remedies, particularly increasing fluid intake, dietary modifications, and using simple analgesics was emphasised. The value of steam in respiratory infection was mentioned.

One effect of this strategy was that more time became available for more serious illnesses and more patients.

When medical resources are scarce and people poor, teaching non-professionals about health may be the only way that the doctor can effectively help his patients. David Werner, who is concerned with providing medical care for 10,000 people in Western Mexico for about one dollar per head per year, commented: 'I began by making a common mistake, that is, trying to provide care instead of helping people to care for themselves.' At his health centre villagers are trained for two months in practical preventive and curative medicine. Some learn to do simple eye surgery, like removing cataracts, others become excellent dentists. From his experience David Werner concludes that medicine itself needs a conceptual shift. Frequently medical students who came to help him boxed themselves into self-erected problem traps. The only escape was to shift from practising medicine to providing care.

The requirement for a conceptual shift in medicine does not only apply to the care of the poor and underprivileged; it is a general need. John McKinlay sees parallels between the development of American medical care and American cars. Fifty years ago cars were '90 per cent transport and 10 per cent frills.' But as Henry Ford discovered, there was not much money in the sort of auto any hick up a country road can keep running with a couple of spanners, and so the car was developed. 'Today a car is 10 per cent transport and 90 per cent frills and most people can't tell what's essential and what isn't. The same has happened to medical care.'

Expectations of medicine have been subject to a long process of over-inflation by the media and the medical profession, as well as by the pharmaceutical industry. It is a process with potentially dangerous consequences. At worst these include the widely held belief that lethal mechanisms we set in motion through our own actions can be reversed. The most common examples of this are the popularly held views that cancer and heart disease may be cured by medical intervention, thus the harmful effects of environmental pollution and cigarette smoking can be safely ignored.

Like other aspects of technology, drugs allow us to distance ourselves from a reality that we are unwilling to confront. We try to avoid the evidence of our mortality. Today we offload the reality onto the doctor, yesterday we used priests, and before that, gods. The doctor's offering of a blessing is in the form of prescribed cotton wool for body and mind. In 1977 Valium was said to be taken by 14 per cent of the population in Britain, the United States and West Germany, 15 per cent in Denmark, and 17 per cent in Belgium and France.[10]

The attitudes of consumers towards drugs are created and maintained by the penetration of the drug industry into all branches of the media. This was strikingly illustrated by an article which appeared in one of Britain's more radical weeklies, the *New Statesman*. The article, entitled 'The Beta Blockade', complained of the refusal by the British Department of Health and Social Security to allow Ciba-Geigy permission to carry out a clinical trial with their beta-blocker oxprenolol (Trasicor). The trial was to assess the suitability of the drug for use of those persons who, through sheer nervousness, are unable to pass their driving tests. 'Even,' the writer claimed, 'although the beneficial effects of beta-blockers on such disparately-stressed citizens as airline pilots, racing drivers, musicians, surgeons and public speakers are well known.'[11] The splendidly irresponsible writer then goes on to describe the entirely beneficial effects of the drug upon her friends and herself while playing music.

Some sense was introduced into this promotional exercise by the drug manufacturer who presumably wished to avoid the more embarrassing implications of the article. 'A spokesman for the manufacturers, Ciba-Geigy, thought that one explanation for the refusal to allow clinical trials might be that the authorities would consider its use in driving tests a trival use for a major drug.' It may also be that the DHSS was aware of the dangers of allowing drugs to be used in this way.

The article is an example of the regrettable nonsense about drugs which appear in large amounts in all media. The damage caused by such material is in the effects it has upon people's attitudes towards the use of drugs. A by-product is the distortion of objectivity in the media themselves, to the point where objective information on drugs is just not available to the general public. Apart from a limited number of books the consumer has no dependable source of objective information in a readily usable form.

Such information could make an enormous contribution both to education and to rational drug use through the universal adoption of the Patient Package Insert (PPI).[12] The arguments for including PPI's in all drugs are basic; to use drugs properly, people need information on their application, and details of likely adverse reactions and side-effects. PPI's enable consumers to make informed choices about their therapy. They have been consistently opposed by the medical establishment. In America the AMA took years finally to agree to the principle of PPI's; in Britain the BMA is still firmly opposed to them.

Anxiety about PPI's usually centres around the wisdom of sharing specific information about adverse reactions and warnings with patients. When the effects of detailed PPI's have been monitored, it has been found that the compliance with therapeutic regimes is not reduced, but patients prefer to have more details. Ninety-five per cent of patients in one study said that they would like PPI's with all drugs.

Until this sort of information is universally available, it is certainly desirable that each household has access to a drug reference source. There are numerous books of this sort, listing drugs, their uses and the major known problems associated with them. Ones we liked are *Medicines: A Guide for Everybody* by Peter Parish (Penguin Books) and *The People's Pharmacy* by Joe Graedon (St Martin's Press).

Despite the profligate misuse of medical resources in the developed world, for the majority of people born on this planet life-long health is a meaningless aspiration. Survival is the simple aim. There are just too many of us, and numbers continue to grow in a way that must always outstrip our capacity to sustain and care. At the corner of Connecticut Avenue and 18th Street in Washington DC, there is a world population indicator. On 21st April 1980, at 10.25 am, it read 4,509,075,595. Each minute 172 was added to the total, representing the net increase when deaths had been subtracted from births. Ten years earlier, the net increase shown on a similar display at the Euvalon in Eindhoven, Netherlands, had been 60 per minute.

In Chapter 5 we noted that among prisoners, high blood pressure was a direct function of the amount of space each inmate had. There is no reason to believe that this process of symptomatic debilitation is not at work in society at large, a threshold contributor to the stress of modern living, which we assume we are powerless to avoid. Not that stress is always bad: large numbers of people, particularly the young, would choose to live in the high static critical mass of large cities with their excitement and opportunity. But the price to be paid for the advantages of such environments is constantly increasing.

Under pressure of numbers, modern life becomes more ordered, more civilised. In the process many of our natural reactions work against us, such as our response to fear. In the wild, fear is an alarm reaction which primes us for fight or flight, whichever gives the best chance of survival. But civilisation puts a brake on these reactions, and instead of adrenalin-primed action, we go into a state of anxiety. We seethe in a world we no longer understand, accepting its novelties and rewards, but paying the price in neurosis and ill-defined stress. The consequent pursuit of relief from life is a generalised phenomenon. American patients, who have to pay, consult doctors just as often as British patients who have free medicine. The economics of the situation seem much less important than other factors; whatever the cost, we seek help with life problems via medicine. This pursuit of an impossible answer inevitably leads to iatrogenic disease.[13]

The alternative to joining the iatrogenic trail is to adopt more positive attitudes towards health. Inevitably this will mean not only changes in outlook, but also changes in habits and lifestyle. The first step may be to accept preventive regimes as a preferable substitute for crisis care. Next, to be rational and realistic about our reliance on current medical systems. This is not a plea for 'alternative medicine', which is notorious for fads and fancies that do not stand the test of time, but more as an encouragement to know ourselves better and understand what can be done to maintain ourselves as healthier individuals. Doctors have made the mistake of treating people as identical mechanical beings; as individuals we must avoid this error.

In most countries the proportion of the health care budget devoted to education is pathetically small, amounting to no more than a token gesture. What resources there are tend to be devoted towards persuading children to avoid bad habits such as smoking and eating junk food, and to pick up elementary hygiene. The Saturday morning TV messages, delivered by the cartoon heroes, like 'Hey! Don't be a YUK mouth!', and 'All you really are is what you eat', may make up in impact what they lack in erudition.

But the problem of health education may be more profound than the limited resources and minimal priority it receives. According to Carolyn Russell, Co-ordinator of the Blue Cross/Blue Shield Health Education Centre in New York, lack of money is not the main obstacle to their work. It is that 'we have no language for health; this is our biggest problem.'

Nevertheless, in the rich nations of the developed world we do have choices about our health. We can choose not to smoke cigarettes, and immediately reduce respiratory infections, cardiovascular problems and lung and other cancers. We can choose a sensible diet and stay around our ideal body weight, and immediately reduce our risks of heart disease and diabetes, as well as improving our general health. We can choose to be physically active, to make our muscles work regularly, and do more with our lives. We can make choices about our environment, both personal and political. We can move to climates and cultures that suit us, and we can insist on the preservation of a healthy, unpolluted environment.

We can also have greater control over our bodily and mental processes than most of us think.[14] A mental determination to fight cancer leads to a higher remission rate than passive acceptance, and strenuous exercise can adjust brain chemistry to counter depression. These are the sort of controls traditionally associated with yoga and meditation, and research into meditation and into biofeedback has confirmed that people can regulate the systems controlled by the autonomic system.

However far we pursue the mechanisms of health into the process of the body and mind, and irrespective of our ability to control or change them, the fundamental determinants of health remain unaltered. Health requires that we be adequately fed, that we be protected from a wide range of hazards in our environment, and that we do not depart radically from the pattern of personal behaviour under which we have evolved. These lessons had been learned by the end of the nineteenth century, and their practical application marked the decline of the major infectious diseases.

This decline can only be adversely affected by the change in emphasis in health care away from environmental and lifestyle factors and towards concepts of 'care' which ignore the importance of cause. Medical care can assist when we become *unavoidably* ill, but it cannot prevent us becoming ill, nor can we rely upon it to provide a cure.

Societies as a whole make choices about the application of resources for the benefit of the population. In choosing chemotherapy, we have been led into a *cul de sac*. Our acceptance of the assumptions and illusions of its benefit has caused us to ignore the fundamental determinants of health. We must retreat and re-think before any further progress can be made.

References

Chapter 1 Consider the Possibility

1 Lawrence, D.R., and Black, J.W., *The Medicine You Take*, London, Croom Helm, 1978.
2 The Sunday Times Insight Team, *Suffer the Children: the Story of Thalidomide*, London, Deutsch, 1979.
3 Wells, N., *Medicines: 50 Years of Progress 1930–1980*, London, Office of Health Economics, 1980.
4 Silverman, M., and Lee, P.R., *Pills, Profits and Politics*, Berkeley, University of California Press, 1974.
5 Brewer, C., 'Medical Miscellany', *General Practitioner*, 25th May 1979, p. 22.
6 *Scrip 408*, 1st August 1979, p. 3.
7 Committee of Principal Investigators, 'A co-operative trial in the primary prevention of ischaemic heart disease using clofibrate', *British Heart Journal*, *401*, 1978, 1069–1118.
8 Teeling-Smith, G., speaking on BBC Radio 4, 4th September 1979.
9 Concerned Rush Students, *A Critical Look at the Drug Industry*. New York: Health Policy Advisory Center.
10 Lang, R.W., *The Politics of Drugs*, Farnborough, Saxon House, 1974.
11 Silverman and Lee, *op. cit.*
12 Martin, E.W., Opening statement, DIA/AMA/FDA/PMA joint symposium, 'Drug information for patients', *Drug Information Journal*, *11*, Special Supplement, January 1977, 2S–3S.
13 Brodie, D.C., *Drug Utilization and Drug Utilization Review and Control*, United States Department of Health, Education and Welfare, National Center for Health Services Research and Development, 1970, p. 2.
14 Melville, A., 'The influence of general practitioners' attitudes on their prescribing', in D. Oborne, M. Gruneberg and J.R. Eiser (eds.), *Research in Psychology and Medicine*, London, Academic Press, 1980.

Chapter 2   Seduced by an Idea

1   Hemminki, E., 'The role of prescriptions in therapy', *Medical Care, 13*, 1975, 150–59.
2   Quoted in Diesendorf, M. *The Magic Bullet*, Canberra, Society for Social Responsibility in Science, 1976.
3   Levine, R.R. *Pharmacology: Drug Actions and Reactions*, Boston, Little, Brown, 1978.
4   Lawrence, D.R., and Black, J.W., *The Medicine You Take*, London, Croom Helm, 1978.
5   Levine, *op. cit.*
6   Vale, J.A., 'Paediatric Poisoning', *Prescribers' Journal, 18*, June 1978, p. 69.
7   Prescott, L.., 'Mechanisms of toxicity – specific therapy', A.M. Breckenridge (ed.), *Advanced Medicine: Topics in Therapeutics*, Tunbridge Wells, Pitman Medical, 1975.
8   Lawrence and Black, *op. cit.*
9   Wade, O.L., *Adverse Reactions to Drugs*, London, Heinemann, 1970.
10   Quoted in Laurence and Black, *op. cit.*
11   Lawson, D., 'Intensive monitoring – the Boston Collaborative Drug Surveillance Program', Inman, W. (ed.), *Monitoring for Drug Safety*, Lancaster, MTP Press, 1980, pp. 213–33.
12   McIntyre, J., 'Pill usage slumps 10pc', *General Practitioner*, 1979.
13   Mapes, R.E.A., 'Physicians' drug innovation and relinquishment', *Social Science and Medicine, 11*, 1977, 619–24.
14   Lawrence and Black, *op. cit.*
15   Skegg, D.C.G., Medical Record Linkage, Inman (ed.), *op. cit.*, p. 337.
16   Price-Evans, D.A., 'Genetic factors in adverse drug reactions', Inman (ed.), *op. cit.*, p. 315.
17   Laurence and Black, *op. cit.*
18   *Ibid.*
19   Wade, *op. cit.*
20   'Side effects of practolol', leader, *British Medical Journal*, 14th June, 1975.
21   Dalton, K., *The Premenstrual Syndrome and Progesterone Therapy*, London, Fontana, 1978.
22   Smithells, R.W., 'Drug Teratogenicity', Inman (ed.), *op. cit.*, p. 307.
23   Sunday Times Insight Team, *Suffer the Children: the story of thalidomide*, London, Deutsch, 1979.
24   Greenberg, G., Inman, W.H.W., Weatherall, J.A.C., Adelstein, A.M., and Haskey, J.C., 'Maternal drug histories and congenital abnormalities', *British Medical Journal*, 1st October 1977, 853–6.
25   Lawrence and Black, *op. cit.*
26   Lawson, *op. cit.*, p. 234.
27   Richards, P., 'Drug-induced metabolic disease', *British Medical Journal, 1*, 1979, 1128–29.
28   Melville, A., and Mapes, R., 'Anatomy of a disaster', Mapes, R. (ed.), *Prescribing Practice and Drug Usage*, London, Croom Helm, 1980, pp. 121–44.
29   Mapes, R.E.A., *op. cit.*
30   Quoted in Diesendorf, *op. cit.*

Chapter 3 Qualified Success

1 Silverman, M., and Lee, P.R., *Pills, Profits and Politics*, Berkeley, University of California Press, 1974, p. 258.
2 Hinman, E.H., *World Eradication of Infectious Diseases*, Springfield, Ill., Charles C. Thomas, 1966.
3 Wilson, D., *Penicillin in Perspective*, London, Faber & Faber, 1976.
4 Hinman, *op. cit.*
5 *Ibid.*
6 Wilson, *op. cit.*
7 *Ibid.*
8 *Scrip 598*, 10th June 1981, p. 9.
9 McKinlay, J., and McKinlay, S., 'The questionable contribution of medical measures to the decline of mortality in the United States in the twentieth century', *Millbank Memorial Fund Quarterly*, 1977, 405–28.
10 McKeown, T., *The Role of Medicine: Dream, Mirage, or Nemesis?*, Oxford, Oxford University Press, 1976.
11 Stewart, G.T., 'Vaccination against whooping-cough: efficacy versus risks', *Lancet*, 29 January 1977, 234–7.
12 Stewart, G.T., 'Toxicity of pertussis vaccine: frequency and probability of reactions', *Journal of Epidemiology and Community Health*, 1979, *33*, 150–56.
13 *Scrip 600*, 17th June 1981, p. 6.
14 *Scrip 605*, 6th July, 1981, p. 3.
15 Wilson, *op. cit.*
16 *Ibid.*
17 *Ibid.*
18 Smith, H., *Antibiotics in Clinical Practice*, London, Pitman Medical, 1977.
19 Wilson, *op. cit.*
20 Smith, *op. cit.*
21 Wilson, *op. cit.*
22 Smith, *op. cit.*
23 Dunlop, Sir D., *Medicines in Our Time*, The Rock Carling Fellowship, The Nuffield Hospitals Trust, 1973, p. 9.
24 Lawrence, D.R., and Black, J.W., *The Medicine You Take*, London, Croom Helm, 1978.
25 West, K.M., *Epidemiology of Diabetes and its Vascular Lesions*, New York, Elsevier, 1978.
26 Quoted from Lawrence, R.D., *The Diabetic Life* (1925), in Lawrence and Black, *op. cit.*
27 Malins, J.M., 'Causes of death in diabetics', Duncan, L.J.P. (ed.), *Diabetes Mellitus*, Edinburgh University Press, 1966.
28 Fink, M., *Convulsive Therapy: Theory and Practice*, New York, Raven Press, 1979.
29 Lawrence and Black, *op. cit.*
30 Cochrane, A.L., and Moore, F., 'Expected and observed values for the prescription of vitamin B_{12} in England and Wales', *British Journal of Preventive and Social Medicine*, *25*, 1971, 147–51.
31 Cole, F., *Milestones in Anaesthesia*, Lincoln, University of Nebraska Press, 1965.
32 Wilson, A., Schild, H.O., and Modell, W., *Applied Pharmacology*, New York, Churchill Livingstone, 1975.

33   Lawrence and Black, *op. cit.*
34   Cole, *op. cit.*
35   Wells, N., *Medicines: 50 Years of Progress 1930–1980*, London, Office of Health Economics, 1980.
36   *New England Journal of Medicine*, 1981, *304*, 801.
37   *Scrip 636*, 21st October 1981, p. 11.
38   Trafford, J.A.P., Horn, C.R., O'Neal, H., McGonigle, R., Halford-Maw, L., and Evans, R., 'Five year follow-up of effects of treatment of mild and moderate hypertension', *British Medical Journal*, *282*, 1981, 1111–13.
39   Wells, *op. cit.*
40   *Scrip 616*, 12th August 1981, p. 16.
41   *Scrip 570*, 4th March 1981, p. 14.
42   Committee on Safety of Medicines, *Current Problems*, No. 6, July 1981.
43   Wyllie, J.H., Clark, C.G., Alexander-Williams, J., Bell, P.R.F., Kennedy, T.L., Kirk, R.M., MacKay, C., 'Effect of cimetidine on surgery for duodenal ulcer', *Lancet*, 18th June 1981, 1307–8.
44   Bardham, K.D., and Hinchcliffe, R.F.C., 'Effect of cimetidine on surgery for duodenal ulcer' (letter), *Lancet*, ii, 4th July 1981, 38.
45   Dunlop, Sir D., *op. cit.* p. 12.

Chapter 4   The Medicine Men

1   Coleman, V., *The Medicine Men*, London, Temple Smith, 1975.
2   *Ibid.*, p. 18.
3   *Ibid.*, p. 20.
4   Lang, R.W., *The Politics of Drugs*, Farnborough, Saxon House, 1974.
5   Chesher, G., M. Diesendorf (ed.), *The Magic Bullet*, Canberra, Society for Social Responsibility in Science, 1976.
6   Cooper, M.H., *Prices and Profits in the Pharmaceutical Industry*, London, Pergamon Press, 1966.
7   Coleman, *op. cit.*
8   Lang, *op. cit.*, p. 19.
9   Barnhart, R., *The Medical Profession-Drug Industry Alliance*, Appendix A, Tufts University School of Medicine, Boston Student Health Organisation, 1970.
10   Tugendhat, C., *The Multinationals*, Harmondsworth, Pelican, 1973.
11   Coleman, *op. cit.*
12   Hearings before the Subcommittee on Monopoly, Select Committee on Small Business, United States Senate, Part 12.
13   Lang, *op. cit.*
14   Silverman, M., and Lee, P.R., *Pills, Profits and Politics*, Berkeley, University of California Press, 1974.
15   HEW, *Task Force on Prescription Drugs*, Washington, United States Government Printing Office, 1968, p. 19.
16   Silverman and Lee, *op. cit.*, p. 111.
17   Kefauver, quoted by Lang, *op. cit.*
18   Slatter, S. St. P., *Competition and Marketing Strategies in the Pharmaceutical Industry*, London, Croom Helm, 1977.
19   HEW, Task Force Report, *op. cit.*
20   Lang, *op. cit.*

21 Cooperstock, R., *Social Aspects of the Medical Use of Psychotropic Drugs*, Toronto, Alcoholism and Drug Addiction Research Foundation, 1974.
22 Lang, *op. cit.*
23 The Banks Committee, *Report of the Committee to Examine the Patent System and Patent Law*, London, HMSO, 1970, p. 116.
24 *Report of the Committee of Enquiry into the Relationship of the Pharmaceutical Industry with the National Health Service*, (The Sainsbury Report), London, HMSO, Cmnd. 3410, 1967, p. 90.
25 Barnhart, R., *The Drug Industry*, Tufts University School of Medicine, Boston Student Health Organisation, 1970.
26 Lang, *op. cit.*
27 Eaton, G., and Parish, P., 'Sources of Drug Information used by General Practitioners', Parish, P., Stimson, G., and Mapes, R., (eds.), Prescribing in General Practice, *Journal of the Royal College of General Practitioners*, 26, *Supp. 1*, 1976.
28 Data Sheet Compendium, 1981, p. 978.
29 BBC Radio 4, *In Sickness or in Wealth*, 4th September 1979.
30 *Ibid.*
31 Steward, H.F., 'Public policy and innovation in the drug industry', Black, D., and Thomas G.P., (eds.), *Providing for the Health Services*, London, Croom Helm, 1978, pp. 132–53.
32 Marion Finkel, Director, New Drug Evaluation, FDA: interview with authors.
33 HEW, *New Drug Evaluation Project Briefing Book*, 1979.
34 Ledogar, R.J., *Hungry for Profits*, New York, IDOC, 1975.
35 *Scrip 498*, 18th June 1980, p. 2.
36 Concerned Rush Students, *A Critical Look at the Drug Industry*, New York, Health/PAC.
37 Lang, *op. cit.*, p. 60.
38 *Ibid.*, p. 61.
39 *Ibid.*, p. 72.
40 *Ibid.*, p. 76.
41 *Ibid.*
42 *Ibid.*

Chapter 5   Good Business Sense

1 Blum, R., 'Factors affecting individual use of medicines,' Blum, R., Herxheimer, A., Stenzland, C., and Woodcock, J. (eds.), *Pharmaceuticals and Health Policy*, London, Croom Helm, 1981.
2 Silverman, M., and Lee, P.R., *Pills, Profits and Politics*, Berkeley, University of California Press, 1974.
3 Chadduck, H.W., *'In Brief Summary': Prescription Drug Advertising, 1962–71*, Washington, FDA Papers, February 1972 (FDA), 72–3026.
4 Coleman, V., *Paper Doctors: a Critical Assessment of Medical Research*, London, Temple Smith, 1977, p. 98.
5 Wingerson, L., 'Sceptical reception for new asthma drug', *New Scientist, 83*, 707, 6th September 1979.
6 Senate Committee on Small Business, Hearings before the Subcommittee on Monopoly, Part II.

7   *Ibid.*
8   *Scrip 400*, 4th July, 1979, p. 9.
9   Letter from Sidney Wolfe and the Health Research Group to Hon. Patricia Harris, Secretary, HEW, 30th August 1979.
10 Slatter, S. St. P., *Competition and Marketing Strategies in the Pharmaceutical Industry*, London, Croom Helm, 1977.
11 *Ibid.*
12 BBC Radio 4, *In Sickness or in Wealth*, 4th September 1979.
13 Fitzgerald, F., 'Detailmen in white coats', *New England Journal of Medicine*, *301*, 20th September 1979, p. 668.
14 Slatter, *op. cit.*
15 *Ibid.*
16 *Ibid.*
17 Scrip and Stockton Institute, 'World Trends in the Pharmaceutical Industry, 1976–1980', quoted in Slatter, *op. cit.*
18 Gordon, B., 'Prescribing practices and drugs information: problems and prospects', speech published by Health Research Group, Washington.
19 Barnhart, R., *The Medical Profession-Drug Industry Alliance*, Tufts University School of Medicine, Boston Student Health Organisation, 1970.
20 Prichard, B.N.C., 'Collaborating with the pharmaceutical industry', *British Medical Journal*, 17th March 1979, 747.
21 Anderson, E.S., 'The problem and implications of chloramphenicol resistance in the typhoid bacillus', *Journal of Hygiene*, 74, 1975, 289–99.
22 *Report of the Royal Commission on the National Health Service*, London, HMSO, 1979.
23 Slatter, *op. cit.*
24 Silverman, M., Lee, P.R., and Lydecker, M., 'The Drugging of the Third World', *Background Reader for the Tenth IOCU World Congress*, June 1981, The Hague, International Organization of Consumers Unions, 127–31.
25 Silverman, M., and Lydecker, M., 'The promotion of prescription drugs and other puzzles', Blum *et al.* (eds.), *op. cit.*, pp. 78–92.
26 Takahashi, K., and Mizuma, M., 'Recommendations and reports for discussion at the medical workshop', *IOCU, op. cit.*, 92–126.
27 *Ibid.*
28 Yudkin, J., Personal communication.
29 Silverman, M., *The Drugging of the Americas*, Berkeley, University of California Press, 1975.
30 Silverman and Lydecker, *op. cit.*
31 Lang, R.W., *The Politics of Drugs*, Farnborough, Saxon House, 1974.
32 Inglis, B., *Drugs, Doctors and Disease*, London, Mayflower, 1965.
33 *Scrip 511*, 4th August 1980, p. 10.
34 Maynard, R., 'Omaha pupils given "behaviour" drugs', *Washington Post*, 29th June 1980, p. 1.
35 Messinger, E., 'Ritalin and MBD: a cure in search of a disease', New York, *Health/PAC Bulletin*, 67, 1975, 1–21.
36 Hughes, R., and Brewin, R., *The Tranquilizing of America*, New York, Harcourt Brace Jovanovich, 1979.
37 *Ibid.*
38 Messinger, *op. cit.*
39 Sugarman, G.I., and Stone, M.N., *Your Hyperactive Child: a Doctor Answers Parents' and Teachers Questions*, Chicago, Henry Regnery Co., 1974, p. 54.

40 Messinger, *op. cit.*
41 Grant, E.C.G., 'Advances in the management of migraine', *Migraine News,* 35, 1977, 1–3.
42 'Poisoning and enuresis', leader, *British Medical Journal,* 17th March 1979, 785–6.
43 Cronin, A.J., Khalil, R.K., and Little, T.M., 'Poisoning with tricyclic anti-depessants: an avoidable cause of childhood deaths', *British Medical Journal,* 17th March 1979, p. 722.
44 Leader, *op. cit.*
45 Zyma (UK) Ltd, 1978–9 advertising campaign for Paroven (hydroxyethyl-rutosides 250mg).
46 Hughes and Brewin, *op. cit.*
47 *Ibid.*
48 Reilly, M., 'The rise and fall of diverticular disease', *World Medicine,* 21st September 1977, 25–31.
49 *Guardian* (Manchester and London), 1st May 1981, p. 1.
50 Taylor, L., Foster, M.C., and Beevers, D.G., 'Divergent views of hospital staff on detecting and managing hypertension', *British Medical Journal,* 1, 1979, 71.
51 Barber, J.H., Beevers, D.G., Fife, R., Hawthorne, V.M., McKenzie, H.M., Sinclair, R.G., Simpson, R.J., Stewart, G.M., and Williams, D.I., 'Blood pressure screening and supervision in general practice', *British Medical Journal,* 31st March 1979, 843–6.
52 Dworkin, B.R., Filewich, R.U., Miller, N.E., and Craigmayle, N., 'Baroreceptor activation reduces reactivity to noxious stimulation: implications for hypertension', *Science,* 205, 1979, 1299–301.
53 Nixon, P., '"Over the hump" in hypertension', *General Practitioner,* 19th January 1979, 29.
54 Cox, V.C., Paulus, P.B., and McCain, G., 'The relationship between crowding and manifestations of illness in prison settings', Oborne, D., Gruneberg, M., and Eiser, J., (eds.), *Research in Psychology and Medicine,* London, Academic Press, 1980.
55 Nixon, *op. cit.*
56 Morgan, T., Gillies, A., Morgan, G., Adam, W., Wilson, M., and Carney, S., 'Hypertension treated by salt restriction', *Lancet,* 4th February 1978, p. 8058.
57 'Salt and High Blood Pressure', *Consumer Reports,* 1979.
58 Stamler, R., Stamler, J., Riedlinger, W.F., Algara, G., and Roberts, R.H., 'Weight and blood pressure', *Journal of the American Medical Association, 240,* 1978, 1607–10.
59 Ramsay, L.E., Ramsay, M.H., and Hettiarachi, J., *British Medical Journal,* 2, 1978, 244–5.
60 Madias, N., 'What you can do about high blood pressure', *Tufts-New England Medical Center Family Health Guides,* 1978.
61 Carey, R.M., Reid, R.A., Ayers, C.R., Lynch, S.S., McLain, W.L., and Vaughan, E.D., 'The Charlottesville blood-pressure survey', *Journal of the American Medical Association, 236* 1976, 847–51.
62 Page, I.M., 'The continuing failure to understand and treat hypertension', *Journal of the American Medical Association, 241,* 1979, pp. 1897–8.
63 DHSS, *Personal and Social Services Statistics,* London, HMSO, 1978.
64 *Scrip 586,* 29th April, 1981, p. 10.
65 *Scrip 587,* 4th May 1981, p. 3.

66   Norsk Medisinaldepot, *Legemiddel-forbruket i Norge,* Oslo, 1978.
67   *Scrip 628,* 23rd September 1981, p. 9.
68   *Scrip 624,* 9th September 1981, p. 9.
69   Office of Population, Census and Surveys, *Health Trends,* London, HMSO, 1980.
70   *Scrip 572,* 11th March 1981, p. 10.
71   *Scrip 624,* 9th September 1981, p. 2.
72   DHSS, *op. cit.*

Chapter 6   Evidence and Effects

1   Coleman, V., *The Medicine Men,* London, Temple Smith, 1975.
2   Wolfe, S.M., Public Citizen Health Research Group, *Statement before FDA Ob-Gyn Advisory Committee,* 30th January 1978.
3   Sjostrom, H., and Nilsson, R., *Thalidomide and the Power of the Drug Companies,* London, Penguin, 1972.
4   Robinson, D., *The Process of Becoming Ill,* London, Routledge & Kegan Paul, 1971.
5   McKinlay, J., and McKinlay, S., *A Refutation of the Thesis that the Health of the Nation is Improving,* in press, 1979.
6   *Ibid.*
7   McKinlay, J., and McKinlay, S., 'The questionable contribution of medical measures to the decline of mortality in the United States in the twentieth century', *Milbank Memorial Fund Quarterly,* 1977, 405–28.
8   McKeown, T., *The Role of Medicine: Dream, Mirage, or Nemesis?,* Oxford, Oxford University Press, 1976.
9   Lambert, P.M., 'Hypertensive disease, study on mortality', *World Health Organisation Bulletin,* 1975, 401–21.
10   World Health Organisation, *World Health Statistics Annual,* 1978.
11   *Ibid.*
12   DHSS, *Health and Social Services Statistics,* London, HMSO, 1978.
13   *U.S. Statistics Annual,* 1978.
14   Government Statistical Office, *Health Trends,* London, HMSO, 1977.
15   Cochrane, A.L., St Leger, A.S., and Moore, F., 'Health service 'input' and mortality 'output' in developed countries', *Journal of Epidemiology and Community Health,* 1978, 32, 200–205.
16   Comptroller General, report to the Congress of the United States, *Evaluating Benefits and Risks of Obstetric Practices – More Coordinated Federal and Private Efforts Needed,* United States General Accounting Office, 1979.
17   'Profile of Doris Haire – patient advocate', *Medical News,* 4th April 1977.
18   Tew, M., 'Is home a safer place?' *Health and Social Service Journal,* 30th May 1980, 702–5.
19   McKinlay and McKinley, *op. cit.,* 1979.
20   Furness, B., M. Diesendorf (ed.), *The Magic Bullet,* Canberra, Society for Social Responsibility in Science, 1976.
21   *United Nations Statistics Annual,* 1978.
22   *Scrip 561,* 2nd February 1981, p. 12.
23   *Scrip 628,* 23rd September 1981, p. 9.
24   DHSS, *op. cit.*
25   Dawson, A.A., 'Drug-induced haematological disease', *British Medical*

Journal, 1, 1979, pp. 1195–7.
26 'The Adrenal Glands', *Update*, 15th September 1979, 793–602.
27 DHSS, *op. cit.*
28 FDA Commisioner Ley, quoted in *Science*, 29th August 1969, p. 877.
29 Ruskin, A., and Anello, C., 'The USA', Inman, W. (ed.), *Monitoring for Drug Safety*, Lancaster, MTP Press, 1980, p. 85.
30 Jick, H., Miettenin, O.S., Shapiro, S., Lewis, G.P., Siskind, V., and Slone, D., 'Comprehensive drug surveillance', *Journal of the American Medical Association, 213*, 1970, 1455.
31 Smith, J.W., Seidl, L.G., and Cluff, L.E., 'Studies on the epidemiology of adverse drug reactions, V. Clinical factors influencing susceptibility', *Annals of Internal Medicine, 65*, 1966, 629.
32 Moir, D., 'Intensive monitoring in hospitals, II: The Aberdeen-Dundee system, Inman (ed.), *op. cit.*, 241.
33 Silverman, M., and Lee, P.R., *Pills, Profits and Politics*, Berkeley, University of California Press, 1974.
34 Melmon, K.L., 'Preventable drug reactions', quoted in Silverman and Lee, *op. cit.*
35 Shapiro, S., Slone, D., Lewis, G.R., and Jick, H., 'Fatal drug reactions among medical inpatients', *Journal of the American Medical Association, 216*, 1971, 467.
36 *Ibid.*
37 Editorial, 'Diseases Drugs Cause', *New England Journal of Medicine, 279*, 1968, p. 1286.
38 Maguire, G.P., Tait, A., Brooke, M., Thomas, C., Howat, J.M.T., Sellwood, R.A., and Bush, H., 'Psychiatric morbidity and physical toxicity associated with adjuvant chemotherapy after mastectomy', *British Medical Journal*, 1st November 1980, 1179–80.
39 Martys, C.R., 'Adverse reactions to drugs in general practice', *British Medical Journal*, 2, 1979, pp. 407–10.
40 *Scrip 418*, 5th September 1979.
41 Wolfe, S.M., 'Testimony before the Senate health subcommittee on adverse consequences of overprescribed drugs', 25th February 1974.
42 Mapes, R.E.A., and Williams, W.O., 'Changes in prescribing patterns, 1970 to 1975', *Journal of the Royal College of General Practitioners*, 1979, 29, 406–12.
43 British Medical Association and the Pharmaceutical Society, *The British National Formulary*, 1976–8.
44 DHSS, *op. cit.*
45 'Drugs and male sexual function', leader, *British Medical Journal*, 1979, 2, 883–4.
46 Castleman, M., 'The sperm crisis', *Medical Self Care*, 8, Spring 1980.
47 Lee, B., and Turner, W., 'Food and Drug Administration's adverse drug reaction monitoring program', *American Journal of Hospital Pharmacy, 25*, 1978, 929–32.
48 The Medicines Commission, *Annual Report for 1978*, London, HMSO.
49 Girdwood, R.H. 'Death after taking medicaments', *British Medical Journal*, 1974, 1, 501–4.
50 Inman, W.H.W., and Adelstein, A.M., 'Rise and fall of asthma mortality in England and Wales in relation to use of pressurised aerosols', *Lancet*, 1969, 2, 279–85.
51 Skegg, D.C.G., Richards, S.M., and Doll, R., 'Minor tranquillisers and road

accidents', *British Medical Journal*, 1979, 1.

52 Editorial, *New England Journal of Medicine*, 26th July 1979, 215.

53 Lennard, H.L., Epstein, L.J., Bernstein, A., and Ransom, D.C., *'Mystification and Drug Misuse'*, San Francisco, Jossey-Bass, 1971.

54 Vorhees, C.V., Brunner, R.L., and Butcher, R.E., 'Psychotropic drugs as behavioural teratogens', *Science*, 205, 1979, 1220–25.

55 Kolata, G.B., 'Behavioural teratology: birth defects of the mind', *Science*, 202, 1978, 732–4.

56 Preston, *Mortality Patterns in National Populations*, London, Academic Press, 1976.

57 Martin, E.W., Opening statement, DIA/AMA/FDA/PMA joint symposium, 'Drug information for patients', *Drug Information Journal*, 11, Special Supplement, January 1977, 2S–3S.

Chapter 7   Guardian Angels

1 Teeling-Smith, G., and Wells, N., Introduction, *Medicines for the year 2000*, London, Office of Health Economics, 1979.

2 Department of Health, Education and Welfare, *New Drug Evaluation Project Briefing Book*, HEW, Rockville, 1979.

3 Laurence, D., and Black, J., *The Medicines You Take*, London, Croom Helm, 1978.

4 Interview with Bill Purvis, Division of Drug Advertising, FDA.

5 HEW, *op. cit.*

6 'Preclinical and clinical testing by the pharmaceutical industry', *Joint Hearings before the subcommittee on Health of the Committee on Labor and Public Welfare and the Subcommittee on Administrative Practice and Procedure of the Committee on the Judiciary*, United States Senate, 94th Congress, 2nd Session, Part II, January 1976.

7 Lambert, E.C., *Modern Medical Mistakes*, Bloomington, Indiana University Press, 1978, p. 86.

8 Sjostrom, H., and Nilsson, A., *Thalidomide and the Power of the Drug Companies*, London, Penguin, 1972.

9 Horita, A., and Hill, H.F., 'Hallucinogens, amphetamines and temperature regulation', *The Pharmacology of Thermoregulation*, Basel, Karger, 1972.

10 Judith Jones, Director, Division of Drug Experience, FDA; personal communication.

11 The Sunday Times Insight Team, *Suffer the Children*, London, Deutsch, 1979.

12 Gill, W.B., Schumacher, G.F.B., Bibbo, M., and Straws, F.H., 'Association of diethylstilboestrol exposure in utero with cryptorchidism, testicular hypoplasia, and semen abnormalities', *Journal of Urology*, 122, (1) 1979, 36–9.

13 Frances Kelsey, Director, Bio-Research Monitoring Program: interview.

14 Holden, C., 'FDA tells Senators of doctors who fake data in clinical drug trials', *Science*, 296, 26th October 1979, 432–3.

15 Committee of Principal Investigators, 'A co-operative trial in the primary prevention of ischaemic heart disease using clofibrate', *British Heart Journal*, 40, 1978, 1069–1118.

16 Committee of Principal Investigators, 'W.H.O. co-operative trial on primary prevention of ischaemic heart disease using clofibrate to lower serum cholesterol: mortality follow-up', *Lancet*, 23rd August 1980, 379–85.

17 *Guardian* (London and Manchester), 21st August 1980.
18 The Anturane Reinfarction Trial Research Group, 'Sulfinpyrazone in the prevention of sudden death after myocardial infarction', *New England Journal of Medicine, 302*, 1980, pp. 250–56.
19 Temple, R., and Pledger, G.W., 'Special Report: The FDA's critique of the Anturane reinfarction trial', *New England Journal of Medicine, 305*, 1980, 488–92.
20 Jones, J.K., 'Assessment of adverse drug reactions in the hospital setting: considerations', *Hospital Formulary, 14*, 1978, pp. 769–76.
21 *Ibid.*
22 Jones, J.K., *The FDA's Adverse Reaction Reporting Program*, Washington, HEW, 1979.
23 Slone, D., Shapiro, S., Kaufman, D.W., Rosenberg, L., Miettinen, O.S., and Stolley, P.D., 'Risk of myocardial infarction in relation to current and discontinued use of oral contraceptives', *New England Journal of Medicine, 305*, 1980, 420–24.
24 Kolata, G.B., 'The phenformin ban: Is the drug an imminent hazard? *Science, 203*, 1979, pp. 1094–6.
25 Knapp, D.E., Zax, B.B., Rossi, A.C., and O'Neill, R.T., 'A method for post-marketing screening of adverse reactions to drugs: Initial results', *Drug Intelligence and Clinical Pharmacy, 14*, 1980, 23–7.
26 *Ibid.*
27 The Medicines Commission, *Annual Report for 1978*. London, HMSO, 1979.
28 Marion Finkel, Director, New Drug Evaluation, FDA: interview.
29 Lunde, I., paper given to British Institute of Regulatory Affairs, reported in *Scrip 462*, 13th February 1980, p. 2.
30 Denis Cahal, DHSS, interview.
31 Coleman, V., *The Medicine Men*, London, Temple Smith, 1975.
32 The Medicines Commissions, *Ibid.*
33 *Scrip 557*, 19th January 1981, p. 4.
34 Inman, W.H.W., 'Postmarketing surveillance of adverse drug reactions in general practice I: search for new methods', *British Medical Journal, 282*, 1981, pp. 1131–2.
35 Inman, W.H.W., 'Detection and investigation of adverse drug reactions', D.M. Davies (ed.), *Textbook of Adverse Drug Reactions*, Oxford, Oxford University Press, 1977, pp. 41–53.
36 *Ibid.*
37 Melville, A., and Mapes, R., 'Anatomy of a disaster: the case of practolol', Mapes, R. (ed.), *Prescribing Practice and Drug Usage*, London, Croom Helm, 1980, pp. 121–44.
38 Wolfe, S., and the Health Research Group, letter to Hon. Patricia Harris, Secretary, HEW, 30th August 1979.
39 *Ibid.*
40 *Scrip 462*, 13th February 1980, p. 8.
41 Wolfe, *op. cit.*
42 Inman, W.H.W., and Adelstein, A.M. 'Rise and fall of asthma mortality in England and Wales in relation to use of pressurised aerosols', *Lancet, 2*, 1969, 279–85.
43 *Ibid.*
44 *Ibid.*
45 *Scrip 432*, 24th October 1979, p. 2.

46   *Scrip 423*, 22nd September 1979, p. 11.
47   *Scrip 401*, 7th July 1979, p. 11.
48   Wardell, W., Hassar, M., Anavekar, S.N., and Lasagna, L., 'The rate of development of new drugs in the United States, 1963 through 1975', *Clinical Pharmacology and Therapeutics, 24*, 1978, 133–45.
49   *Newsweek*, 8th January 1973.
50   Nelson, G. statement before the Subcommittee on Monopoly of the Select Committee on Small Business on competitive problems in the drug industry, p. 9107, 1973.
51   Bill Inman, interview.
52   Wolfe, S., and the Public Citizen Health Research Group, letter to FDA Commissioner Jere Goyan, 24th January 1980.
53   Inman, *op. cit.*, 1977.
54   Lang, R.W., *The Politics of Drugs*, Farnborough, Saxon House, 1974.

Chapter 8   Keep on Taking the Tablets

1   'Side effects of practolol', leading editorial, *British Medical Journal*, 14 June 1975, 577.
2   Wright, R. 'Untoward effects associated with practolol administration: oculo-mucocutaneous syndrome', *British Medical Journal*, 1975, 1, 595–8.
3   Raftery, E.B., and Denman, A.M., 'Systemic lupus erythematosus syndrome induced by practolol', *British Medical Journal*, 1973, 2, 452–5.
4   *Ibid.*
5   Hardie, R.A., and Savin, J.A. 'Drug-induced skin diseases', *British Medical Journal*, 7th April 1979, 1, 935–7.
6   Clothier, C.M., and Crawford, P., *Joint Opinion in the Matter of Practolol (Eraldin)*, 1976.
7   Rowland, M.G.M., and Stevenson, C.J., letter, *Lancet*, 1, 1972, p. 1130.
8   Felix, R., and Ive, F.A., 'Skin reactions to practolol' *British Medical Journal*, 11th May 1974, 333.
9   Wright, P., 'Skin reactions to practolol', *British Medical Journal*, 8th June, 1974, 560.
10 Melville, A., and Mapes, R.E.A., 'Anatomy of a disaster', Mapes (ed.), *Prescribing Practice and Drug Usage*, London, Croom Helm, 1980.
11 Clothier and Crawford, *op. cit.*, p. 26.
12 Halley, W., and Goodman, J.D.S. (letter), *British Medical Journal*, 2, 1975, 337.
13 Eraldin Action Group/Community Health Council estimate.
14 Clothier and Crawford, *op. cit.* p. 1.
15 *Ibid.*,
16 Alexander, Tatnam & Co., Blair Allison & Co., Irwin Mitchell & Co., *Eraldin (practolol): Memorandum for the Use of Claimaints' Solicitors.*
17 Chalmers, T., 'Epidemiological surveillance in perinatal practice', Colombo, F., Shapiro, S., Slone, D., and Tognoni, G. (eds.), *Epidemiological Evaluation of Drugs*, Littleton, Mass., PSG Publishing Co. Inc., 1977, pp. 249–55.
18 Wolfe, S., *Sex Hormones Used in Pregnancy and Birth Defects: Another Thalidomide?* Public Citizen Health Research Group, Washington, 1976.
19 Janerich, D.T., Dugan, J.M., Standfast, S.J., and Strite, L., 'Congenital heart disease and prenatal exposure to exogenous sex hormones', *British*

Medical Journal, 1977, 1, 1058–60.
20 Nora, J.J., Nora, A.H., Blue, J., Ingram, J., Fountain, A., Peterson, M., Lortscher, R.M., and Kimberling, W.J., 'Exogenous progestogen and estrogen implicated in birth defects', *Journal of the American Medical Association*, 1978, 240 (9), 837–43.
21 For example see Martindale, *The Extra Pharmacopoeia*, London, The Pharmaceutical Press, 1977.
22 Heinonen, O.P., Slone, D., Monson, R.R., Hook, E.B., and Shapiro, S., 'Cardiovascular birth defects and antenatal exposure to female sex hormones', *New England Journal of Medicine*, 1977, 296, 67–70.

Chapter 9   Everyday Drug Hazards

1 Yudkin, J., 'Provision of medicines in a developing country', *Lancet*, 15th April 1978.
2 Wolfe, S., Testimony before the Senate Health Subcommittee on adverse consequences of overprescribed drugs, 25th February 1974.
3 *Scrip 625*, 14th September 1981, p. 4.
4 *British Medical Journal*, leader, 12th March 1977, 668.
5 Wolfe, S., presentation on Darvon to H.E.W. Secretary Joseph Califano, 31st May 1979.
6 Wolfe, S., testimony before FDA hearings on Darvon, 6th April 1979.
7 Whittington, R.M., 'Dextropropoxyphene (Distalgesic) overdose in the West Midlands', *British Medical Journal*, 16th July 1977, 172–3.
8 *British Medical Journal*, leader, *op. cit.*
9 Martindale, *The Extra Pharmacopaeia*, London, The Pharmaceutical Press, 1977.
10 Vorhees, C.V., Brunner, R.L., and Butcher, R.E., 'Psychotropic drugs as behavioural teratogens', *Science*, 205, 1979, 1220–25.
11 Martindale, *op. cit.*
12 Holdstock, D.J., letter, *Lancet*, 1972, i, 541.
13 Dawson, A.A., 'Drug-induced haematological disease', *British Medical Journal*, 5th May 1979, 1195–7.
14 Martindale, *op. cit.*
15 Knapp, D.E., Zax, B.B., Rossi, A.C., and O'Neill, R.T., 'A method for post-marketing screening of adverse reactions to drugs: initial results', *Drug Intelligence and Clinical Pharmacy*, 14, 1980, 23–7.
16 Frederick, G.R., and Tanaka, K.R., letter, *New England Journal of Medicine*, 1968, 279, 1290.
17 Walls, J., *et al.*, letter, *British Medical Journal*, ii, 1968, 52.
18 Chapman, R.A., *Canadian Medical Association Journal*, 1966, 95, 1156.
19 Kelsey, W.M., & Scharyj, M., *Journal of the American Medical Association*, 1967, 199, 586.
20 Martindale, *op. cit.*
21 Shader, R.I. and DiMascio, A., *Psychotropic drug side effects*, Baltimore, Williams and Wilkins, 1970, pp. 135–6.
22 Parish, P., *Medicines: A Guide for Everybody*, Harmondsworth, Penguin, 1980.
23 Safra, M.J., and Oakley, G.P., 'Association between cleft lip with or without cleft palate and prenatal exposure to diazepam', *Lancet*, 13th September 1975, p. 478.

24   Saxen, I., and Saxen, L., 'Association between maternal intake of diazepam and oral clefts', *Lancet*, ii, 1975, 498.
25   Greenberg, G., Inman, W.H.W., Weatherall, J.A.C., Adelstein, A.M., and Haskey, J.C., 'Maternal drug histories and congenital abnormalities', *British Medical Journal*, 1st October 1977, 853–6.
26   Kellogg, C., Tervo, D., Ison, J., Parisi, T., and Miller, R.K., 'Prenatal exposure to diazepam alters behavioural development in rats', *Science, 207*, 1980, 205–7.
27   Martindale, *op. cit.*
28   Shader and diMascio, *op. cit.*
29   *Ibid.*
30   Martindale, *op. cit.*
31   Greenblatt, D.J., 'Propranolol', Miller, R.R., and Greenblatt, D.J., (eds.), *Drug Effects in Hospitalised Patients: Experiences of the Boston Collaborative Drug Surveillance Program, 1966–1975*, New York, Wiley, 1976.
32   Martindale, *op. cit.*
33   Beller, G.A., *et al.*, *New England Journal of Medicine*, 1971, *284*, 989.
34   Wishner, S.H., *et al.*, *New England Journal of Medicine*, 1972, *287*, 552.
35   Gazes, P.C., *et al.*, *Circulation*, 1961, *23*, 358.
36   Martindale, *op. cit.*
37   Dall, J.L.C., *British Medical Journal*, ii, 1970, 705.
38   Dawson, A., *op. cit.*
39   Toghill, P.J., *et al.*, *British Medical Journal*, iii, 1974, 545.
40   Alexander, W.D., and Evans, J.I., letter, *British Medical Journal*, ii, 1975, 501.
41   Greenblatt, *op. cit.*
42   Martindale, *op. cit.*
43   Parish, *op. cit.*
44   Martindale, *op. cit.*
45   Wolfe, testimony, 1974, *op. cit.*
46   Parish, *op. cit.*
47   Newmark, S.R., 'Ampicillin', Miller & Greenblatt (eds.), *op. cit.*
48   Martindale, *op. cit.*
49   Peters, R.L., *et al.*, *American Journal of Surgery*, 113, 1967, 622.
50   Ribush, N., and Morgan, T., *Medical Journal of Australia*, i, 1972, 53.
51   Martindale, *op. cit.*
52   *Scrip 620*, 26th August 1981, p. 3.
53   Martindale, *op. cit.*
54   Carroll, O.M., *et al.*, *Journal of the American Medical Association*, 195, 1966, 691.
55   Salter, A.J., *Medical Journal of Australia*, i, 30th June 1973, 70.
56   Martindale, *op. cit.*
57   *Ibid.*
58   Goldman, L., and Kitzmiller, W., *Archives of Dermatology*, 107, 1973, 611.
59   Kligman, A.M., and Leyden, J.J., *Journal of the American Medical Association*, 229, 1974, 60.
60   Martindale, *op. cit.*
61   Takahashi, K., and Mizuma, N., 'Recommendations and reports for discussion at the medical workshop', 10th IOCU World Congress, June 1981.
62   Ledogar, R., *Hungry for Profits*, New York, IDOC, 1975.
63   Van der Geest, S., *The Efficiency of Inefficiency: Medicine Distribution in the*

South Camaroon, paper presented at the Seventh International Conference on Social Science and Medicine, Noordwijkerhout, July 1981.

64 Murray, R., 'Side effects of common analgesics', *General Practitioner*, 17th August 1973, 15.

65 Parish, *op. cit.*

66 Lawrence, D.R., and Black, J.W., *The Medicines You Take*, London, Croom Helm, 1978, p. 63.

67 *Ibid.*, p. 64.

68 Davies, A.G., 'The kidney: reducing the risk of drug-related damage', *Modern Medicine*, 17th May 1979, 28–32.

69 Parish, *op. cit.*

70 *Ibid.*

71 Peterson, R.B., and Vasques, L.A., letter, *Journal of the American Medical Association*, 223, 1973, 324.

72 Livingston, P.H., letter, *Journal of the American Medical Association*, 196, 1966, 1159.

73 Duvernoy, W.F.C. *New England Journal of Medicine*, 280, 1969, 877.

74 Martindale, *op. cit.*

75 Parish, *op. cit.*

76 *Ibid.*

Chapter 10   What's Wrong, Doctor?

1 Furnass, B., M. Diesendorf (ed.), *The Magic Bullet*, Canberra, Society for Social Responsibility in Science, 1976, p. 13.

2 Mapes, R., 'Sociological parameters of increased prescribing rate', Mapes, R. (ed.), *Prescribing Practice and Drug Usage*, London, Croom Helm, 1980, pp. 33–6.

3 Johnson, T.J., *Professions and Power*, London, Macmillan, 1972.

4 *Ibid.*

5 Stevens, R., *Medical Practice in Modern England*, New Haven, Yale University Press, 1966.

6 Smith, M.C., 'The relationship between pharmacy and medicine', R. Mapes (ed.), *Prescribing Practice and Drug Usage*, *op. cit.*

7 Cochrane, A., '1931–1971: A critical review, with particular reference to the medical profession', *Medicines for the Year 2000*, London, Office of Health Economics, 1979.

8 Stevens, *op. cit.*

9 Bridgstock, M., *A Sociological Analysis of General Practice Organisation*, unpublished PhD thesis, University College of Swansea, 1978.

10 Chapman, C.B., 'Should there be a commission on medical education?' *Science*, 10th August 1979, 559–62.

11 Larson, M.S., *The Rise of Professionalism: a Sociological Analysis*, Berkeley, University of California Press, 1977.

12 Mapes, R. (ed.) *op. cit.*, Introduction.

13 Dixon, B., *Beyond the Magic Bullet*, London, George Allen & Unwin, 1978.

14 Najman, J.M., and Congleton, A., 'Australian occupational mortality, 1965–67: cause specific or general susceptibility?' *Sociology of Health and Illness*, 1979, *1*, 158–76.

15 Eaton, G., and Parish, P., 'High cost prescribing doctors', in 'Prescribing in

General Practice', *Journal of the Royal College of General Practitioners*, 1976, 26, Supp. 1.

16   Hughes, R., and Brewin, R., *The Tranquilizing of America*, New York, Harcourt Brace Jovanovich, 1979.

17   *Ibid.*

18   Grist, E., 'The medical carapace', *General Practitioner*, 25th May 1979, 42–3.

19   Helfer, R.E., 'An objective comparison of the paediatric interview skills of freshmen and senior medical students', *Paediatrics*, 1970, 45, 623–7.

20   Stimson, G., and Webb, B., *Going To See The Doctor: The Consultation Process in General Practice*, London, Routledge & Kegan Paul, 1975.

21   Sternbach, R. (ed.), *The Psychology of Pain*, New York, Raven Press, 1978.

22   Lennard, H., Epstein, L., Bernstein, A., and Ransom D., *Mystification and Drug Misuse*, San Francisco, Jossey-Bass, 1971.

23   Murray, R.M., 'Psychiatric morbidity among medical practitioners', *Update*, 1st July, 1979, 31–8.

24   Rigler, M., 'The crippling cult of the expert', *General Practitoner*, 17th November 1978, 45.

25   Melville, A., 'Job satisfaction in general practice: implications for prescribing', *Social Science and Medicine*, 14A, 1980, 495–9.

26   Freidson, E., *Profession of Medicine: a Study of the sociology of applied knowledge*, New York, Dodd, Mead, 1970.

27   Melville, A., and Mapes, R., 'Anatomy of a disaster: the case of practolol', Mapes (ed.), *op. cit.*, pp. 121–44.

28   Melville, A., 'The hazards of using prescribing experience', *General Practitioner*, 16th November 1979, 45.

29   Stimson, G.V., 'General practitioners' estimates of patient expectations, and other aspects of their work', Swansea, Medical Sociology Research Centre, Occasional Paper no. 3, 1975.

30   Segal, H.J., 'The social risks and benefits of prescription-writing', Mapes (ed.), *op. cit.*, pp. 19–32.

31   Raynes, N.V., 'What can I do for you?' Mapes (ed.), *op. cit.*, pp. 83–99.

32   Lee, J.A.H., Draper, F.A., and Weatherall, M., 'Primary medical care: prescribing in three English towns', *Millbank Memorial Fund Quarterly*, 1965, 43, 2, 285–90.

33   Joyce, C.R.B., Last, J.M., and Weatherall, M., 'Personal factors as a cause of differences in prescribing by general practitoners', *British Journal of Preventive and Social Medicine*, 1967, 21, 170–77.

34   Smith, M.C., 'The relationship between pharmacy and medicine', Mapes (ed.), *op. cit.*, pp. 157–200.

35   Hall, D., 'Prescribing as social exchange', Mapes (ed.), *op. cit.*, pp. 39–57.

36   Hemminki, E., 'The role of prescriptions in therapy', *Medical Care*, 13, 1975, 150–59.

37   McDevitt,D.G., 'A spoonful of sugar', inaugural lecture, Queen's University of Belfast, 28th February 1979.

38   Heath, C., 'On prescription-writing in social interaction', Mapes (ed.), *op. cit.*, (pre-publication draft).

39   Stimson, G., and Webb, B., *op. cit.*

40   Raynes, N.V., *op. cit.*

41   Hemminki, E., 'The effect of a doctor's personal characteristics and working circumstances on the prescribing of psychotropic drugs', *Medical Care*, 1974, 12, 351–7.

42 Bakwin, R., (1945), quoted in Scheff, T.J., 'Decision rules and their consequences', *Behaviour Science*, 1963, 97–107.
43 Melville, A., 'Reducing whose anxiety? A study of the relationship between
   repeat prescribing of minor tranquillisers and doctors' attitudes', Mapes (ed.),
   op. cit., 100–119.
44 Balint, M., Hunt, J., Joyce, D., Marinker, M., and Woodcock, J., *Treatment
   or Diagnosis*, London, Tavistock, 1970.
45 Becker, M.H., Stolley, P.D., Lasagna, L., McEvilla, J.D., and Sloane,
   L.M., 'Characteristics and attitudes of physicians associated with the prescribing of chloramphenicol', *HSMHA Health Reports*, 1971, 86, 993–1003.
46 Pritchard, P., *Manual of Primary Health Care: Its Nature and Organisation*,
   Oxford, Oxford University Press, 1978.
47 Marks, J.H., Goldberg, D.P., and Hillier, V.F., 'Determinants of the ability
   of general practitioners to detect psychiatric illness', *Psychological Medicine*,
   1979, 9. 337–53.
48 Mapes, R.E.A., 'Physicians' drug innovation and relinquishment', *Social
   Science and Medicine*, 1977, 11, 619–24.
49 Dadja, R., 'The prescribing of General Practitioners in Wales and England – a
   comparison', Swansea, *MSRC, Working Papers on Prescribing No. 4*, 1976.
50 Brewer, C., 'Common medicine in the common market', *General Practitioner*,
   October 12, 1979, 38.
51 Cochrane, A., lecture given at University College of Cardiff, 1980.
52 Norwegian prescribing data from *Norsk Medisinaldepot Legemiddelforbruket i
   Norge*, 1978; UK data from DHSS statistics.

Chapter 11   People As Patients

 1 Dubos, R., *Man, Medicine and Environment*, London, Pall Mall Press, 1968.
 2 Dunnell, K., 'Medicine takers and hoarders', in 'The medical use of psychotropic drugs', *Journal of the Royal College of General Practitioners*, 23, Sup. 2,
   1973, 2–9.
 3 Beecher, H.K., *Measurement of Subjective Responses*, Oxford, Oxford
   University Press, 1959.
 4 Antonovsky, A., *Health, Stress, and Coping*, San Francisco, Jossey-Bass, 1979.
 5 Robinson, D., *The Process of Becoming Ill*, London, Routledge & Kegan Paul,
   1971.
 6 Parsons, T., *The Social System*, London, Routledge & Kegan Paul, 1951.
 7 Fitton, F., and Acheson, H., *The Doctor/Patient Relationship: a Study in
   General Practice*, HMSO, London, 1979.
 8 Cartwright, A., *Patients and Their Doctors: a Study of General Practice*,
   London, Routledge & Kegan Paul, 1967.
 9 *Ibid.*
10 *Ibid.*
11 Stimson, G., and Webb, B., *Going to See the Doctor*, London, Routledge &
   Kegan Paul, 1975.
12 Gregory, S., 'Abdominal tears and the fat note syndrome', *World Medicine*,
   23rd February 1980, 17.
13 Hughes, R., and Brewin, R., *The Tranquilizing of America*, New York,
   Harcourt Brace Jovanovich, 1979, p. 179.

14   Fitzgerald, M., and Sim, J., *British Prisons*, Oxford, Blackwell, 1979. Dr McCleery quoted from *Prison Medical Journal*, p. 111.

Chapter 12   Consultations Like Clockwork

1   Byrne, P.S., and Long, P.E.L., *Doctors Talking to Patients*, London, HMSO, 1976, p. 5.
2   *Ibid.*, p. 9.
3   *Ibid.*, p. 61.
4   *Ibid.*, p. 63.
5   *Ibid.*, p. 116.
6   *Ibid.*, p. 129.
7   *Ibid.*, p. 129.
8   Mechanic, D., *Politics, Medicine and Social Science*, New York, Wiley-Interscience, 1974.
9   Byrne and Long, *op. cit.*, p. 93.
10   Fitton, F., and Acheson, H.W.K., *The Doctor/Patient Relationship: a Study in General Practice*, London, HMSO, 1979, 9. 58.
11   Byrne and Long, *op. cit.*, p. 131.
12   Mulroy, R., 'Iatrogenic disease in general practice: its incidence and effects', *British Medical Journal*, 19th May 1973,. 407–10.
13   *Ibid.*, p. 410
14   Jones, J.K., 'Assessment of adverse drug reactions in the hospital setting: considerations', *Hospital Formulary*, 14, 8, 769–76.
15   Fitton and Acheson, *op. cit.*, p. 80.
16   Byrne and Long, *op. cit.*, p. 59.
17   *Ibid.*, p. 48.

Chapter 13   To Whom Can We Turn?

1   Hughes, R., and Brewin, R., *The Tranquilizing of America*, New York, Harcourt Brace Jovanovich, 1979.
2   Balint, M., Hunt, J., Joyce, D., Marinker, M., and Woodcock, J., *Treatment or Diagnosis?* London, Tavistock, 1970.
3   Bush, D.F., and Carroll, J.G., 'Recent Research on Doctor-Patient Communication in the U.S.A.: Understanding health care interactions and teaching key skills', paper given to the MSD Foundation Colloquium on the Consultation, London, March, 1982.
4   Klein, R., *Complaints Against Doctors: A Study in Professional Accountability*, London, Charles Knight, 1973.
5   Leahy-Taylor, J., 'Medico-legal aspects and implications', D.M. Davies (ed.), *Textbook of Adverse Drug Reactions*, Oxford, Oxford University Press, 1977, pp. 435–45.
6   Cusine, D.J., 'What is medical negligence?', *World Medicine*, 31st May 1980, 21–3.
7   Melville, A., and Mapes, R.E.A., 'Anatomy of a disaster: the case of practolol, Mapes, R. (ed.), *Prescribing Practice and Drug Usage*, London, Croom Helm, 1980.
8   *Scrip 569*, 2nd March 1981, p. 10.

9 Hansson, O., and Herxheimer, A., 'Neuropathy and optic atrophy associated with halquinol', *Lancet*, 21st February 1981, 450.
10 *Scrip 569*, 2nd March 1981, p. 10.
11 Sjostrom, H., and Nilsson, A., *Thalidomide and the Power of the Drug Companies*, Harmondsworth, Penguin, 1972.
12 Medicines Division, DHSS, 'Strict product liability', consultation document.
13 *Scrip 620*, 26th August 1981, p. 3.
14 Hughes and Brewin, *op. cit.*
15 Douglas, D.B., *Experiences in Pills Anonymous*, Unpublished manuscript, Lenox Hill Hospital, New York.

Chapter 14   Possibilities and Perspectives

1 See, for example, Graedon, J., *The People's Pharmacy*, New York, St Martin's Press, 1976.
2 Counter Information Services: CIS Report, *NHS: Condition Critical*, London, CIS, 1980.
3 *Scrip 539*, 10th November 1980, p. 9.
4 *Scrip 564*, 11th February 1981, p. 4.
5 *Scrip 421*, 15th September 1979, p. 3.
6 Eclipse Computer Services, Manchester, Medrisk.
7 Russell, B., *History of Western Philosophy*, London, George Allen and Unwin, 1961.
8 Smith, M.C., 'The relationship between pharmacy and medicine', Mapes, R. (ed.), *Prescribing Practice and Drug Usage*, London: Croom Helm, 1980, p. 194.
9 Marsh, G.N., '"Curing" minor illness in general practice', *British Medical Journal*, 2, 1977, 1267.
10 Coleman, V., *The Medicine Men*, London, Arrow Books, 1977, p. 84.
11 Hall, R., 'The beta blockade', *New Statesman*, 16th March 1979, 354–5.
12 Morris, L.A., 'Rationale for Patient Package Inserts', *American Journal of Hospital Pharmacy*, 35, 1978, 179–84.
13 Illich, I., *Limits to Medicine*, Harmondsworth, Penguin, 1977.
14 Pelletier, K.R., *Mind as Healer, Mind as Slayer*, New York, Dell, 1980.

Index